What We're Told Not to Talk About
(But We're Going to Anyway)

'Hilarious and heartbreaking at the same time, Nimko
has blown apart all taboos . . . Essential reading
for everyone' Scarlett Curtis, author
of *Feminists Don't Wear Pink*

'A beautiful book with such a wide range of
uplifting but often heartbreaking stories. Made us
cry and think in equal measure' Pandora Sykes,
co-host of *The High Low*

'Nimko Ali is a heroine for our time – she
destroys the notion of things being too rude to
discuss' Caitlin Moran, author of *How to Be a Woman*

'*What We're Told Not to Talk About* is going to
shift the conversation around women's
bodies' Amika George, founder of the
Free Periods Campaign

'Nimko says it how it is. There is no subject too
rude for her to tackle. We should all be talking
about our vaginas and she is leading the
way' Bryony Gordon, author of *Mad Girl*

'Nimko Ali is my hero! She's an anti-FGM activist
and is responsible for changing laws across the globe!
She is also hilarious and wonderful' Zoe Sugg (Zoella)

ABOUT THE AUTHOR

Nimko Ali OBE is a feminist, anti-FGM campaigner and professional over-sharer. She is co-founder of The Five Foundation, the global coalition to end FGM. She has been instrumental in changing legislation around the practice of FGM in the UK and abroad, including getting it included in the Children's Act in 2019. She has spoken at events including the Women of the World festival and the Girl Summit. At the 2019 Geneva Summit for Human Rights and Democracy Nimko was awarded the UN Women's Rights Award. *What We're Told Not to Talk About* is her first book.

What We're Told Not to Talk About (But We're Going to Anyway)

Women's Voices from East London to Ethiopia

NIMKO ALI

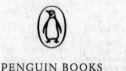

PENGUIN BOOKS

PENGUIN BOOKS

UK | USA | Canada | Ireland | Australia
India | New Zealand | South Africa

Penguin Books is part of the Penguin Random House group of companies
whose addresses can be found at global.penguinrandomhouse.com.

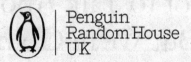

First published by Viking 2019
Published with a new preface in Penguin Books 2020

001

Copyright © Nimko Ali, 2019, 2020

The moral right of the author has been asserted

The publisher is grateful for permission to quote from *Mean Girls* (2004),
reproduced by kind permission of Paramount Pictures.

Every effort has been made to trace copyright holders and to obtain their
permission for the use of copyright material. The publisher apologizes for any
errors or omissions and would be grateful to be notified of any corrections
that should be incorporated in future editions of this book.

Typeset by Jouve (UK), Milton Keynes
Printed and bound in Great Britain by Clays Ltd, Elcograf S.p.A.

A CIP catalogue record for this book is available from the British Library

ISBN: 978-0-241-98760-5

www.greenpenguin.co.uk

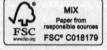

To my Ayeeyo (grandmother): you were and will always be my world. Thank you for always standing up for me and allowing me the freedoms that made me the woman I am today.

I miss you.

Contents

Preface

Since I started writing this book, I have grown so much and I have found a stronger connection between my lived experience and its impact on my fanny and everyday life. As much as we want to deny it, women and girls are very much seen and framed by what they have between their legs and what happens there; it is something we all carry with us every day.

Since the day I was made aware of my anatomy via the brutal act of FGM, thinking about my fanny has consumed me. I used to think I would go mad, and reading some of the journals I wrote in my teen years, I can see I was not okay. As I looked for answers about what had happened to me and what this meant, I found my voice . . . but that was a lonely place.

A place it seems many others also were, and are still, in. Just last week at an international development conference a woman ran up to me to thank me for writing the book her best friend needed as she struggled with pregnancy and motherhood. Like so many young women today, her friend was comparing herself to the media posts of celebs and others who seemed to have it sorted hours after giving birth. She thought she was a failure and could not bring herself to ask for help until she read the stories of women who were honest and open in the book. Many of the emails I get are from women with teenagers thanking me for writing a book they can give to their daughters, and others are from women who are my age and wish they had had this book when we were teens.

This is because sadly, in the nineties and the noughties, people were not as fanny-forward as they are now. The idea of writing a blog, let alone a book, about all the things I wanted to know about the female anatomy was a no-go. I was a first-generation, Muslim, African woman trying to find her feet in a land that was not hers. So, if I did want to talk about women and their privates, it had to be academic.

Yes, I wanted to intellectually masturbate about the issue and to be honest, I thought doing my questing under the remit of academia would be safer. My family would not need to know what I was actually researching, and people would not give me a funny look or get offended when I asked random questions about their vagina or told them about mine. Having read all the research there was on FGM and the female body when growing up, I worked out that none of the information in the books or research papers was first-hand. All the authors were men who did not care as much as a woman would.

This was the era of lad mags so the bar was low when it came to the conversation about the fanny in the media and politics. I wanted to be Nawal El Saadawi, who had saved me in my teens and twenties when I was doing all my thinking in private. Nawal was, and is, an Egyptian feminist activist and a survivor of FGM who wrote powerfully and honestly about the complicated mother-daughter dynamic in her book *The Hidden Face of Eve*. I read her book again and again and these words would be the ones that would shape my life from the age of thirteen:

> I did not know what they had cut off from my body, and I did not try to find out. I just wept and called out to my mother for help. But the worst shock of all was when I looked around and found her standing by my side. Yes, it was her, I could not be mistaken.

I could feel the rage and pain in her words. Like me, she loved her mum, but also blamed her for not saving her and for being part of something horrific. To know that someone out there in the world was not only thinking like me but also writing it down was incredible.

Not feeling alone and connecting to a woman I did not meet till 2014 was amazing and I now know that millions of girls were out there in their bedrooms, bathrooms or wherever they could find the space, thinking about their bodies and experiences but unable to say it out loud. Sadly, this is not the case when it comes to men talking about our bodies: not only did they write all the books, but every single organized religion and culture known to us has had something to say about women and their bodies. So many wars have raged across the world and those raging right now have or will use women's bodies as the battle ground. Others have legislated to control women in one way or another. Women, I was once told by a man, are the objects which men, the subjects, fill up. I know, super gross.

My introduction to my body was an act of violence and something that filled me with fear, which I am just getting to grips with. When I published this book in 2019 I sat on the edge of my bed and cried for hours over the final copy. In the introductions to several chapters I was so honest about so much, I was so open and I was proud of the words I wanted to share with the world. But I was also so scared. I knew that by oversharing and being unapologetic, I was breaking an unspoken rule and showing the power of being free.

I was not ashamed of the sex, periods and possible babies: I wanted to talk about it all. As brave as I seemed to some, those who knew me read my words and worried that I was putting myself in danger. To truly live without shame, especially as a woman like me, is not something I have seen or experienced, but it's something I have been fighting for and it's something I am going to do.

I wrote this book because I wanted to talk about how I first had sex at the age of twenty-one. He was my first boyfriend, even if I did not call him that. In my culture there is no such thing: either you are married or not and to even call a man a 'friend' means you are either fucking him or you want to. I wanted to talk about how I found myself trapped between two cultures and how I felt so terrible, all I could do was cry and cry in a state of guilt and confusion. As a Somali girl, I'd been raised in a religion that said I was not to have sex till I was married, and then I was educated in a Catholic school that taught me the same thing. Pre-marital sex was a sin. I really thought the world was going to end and I was going to die if I had sex outside of marriage. But when I discovered how good sex could be, I soon got over the idea that it was bad and that I needed to feel ashamed. Especially when the other person, who was from the same background as I was, did not feel bad about it.

The feelings of shame and guilt we are consumed by are ones we learn as early as in the womb. To please the woman we came from and to have her acceptance is a task we are all seeking to achieve. It is one I now know is not possible. The death of my grandmother was an eye-opener: it allowed me to see that disappointing the woman who was closest to me was not the end of the world. In fact, it was freedom. To fail in the eyes of your mother and still be happy with the choices you make is the bravest thing you will ever do. I love my mum and I will forever be grateful to her, but I am finally getting to know her as her. I am finding the strength that I wished for as I read Nawal, I am finding the ability to say out loud that my mum is human, she is flawed and that we are two different people. Everything I do will not please her and she will never fully understand me, but we can get on and I don't need to feel bad about not liking her every day.

The prism of the 'Madonna-whore complex' that I have lived in-between for as long as I can remember is finally gone and not because I have become someone else but because I have accepted myself. I can now talk about the ex-boyfriend from LA who would always turn up at the same time as my bloody period (the number of hotel sheets ruined because of his 'I'm too horny to care' attitude runs into the tens). And when I worked out that I could get a week off Ramadan while on my period, I was all about my period. But when I bled for ten days non-fucking-stop when I had the coil fitted, I was happy to have my ovaries removed and be done with this shit.

Writing this and speaking as freely as I have over the last few months is truly liberating, but it's also a work in progress. I have so much more I could, and will, say. I have become very good at being open but also making sure that what I say is not used by those who hate women who are free and able to speak up. When you shake off shame and accept that growth comes with losing some people in your life, you as a woman become the most powerful, which is scary.

Introduction: Fannying About

'For all the feminist progress made, there is still
a shocking amount of disdain for women's
anatomy when it is not firm, tucked,
primped and waxed.'

— Jessica Valenti

Remember that scene in *Mean Girls* when the girls in the school hall are pushed to share issues they are having with other female students, and one girl announces, 'Someone wrote in that book that I'm lying about being a virgin 'cause I use super-jumbo tampons, but I can't help it if I've got a heavy flow and a wide-set vagina.'

The censors had a problem with that line. They wanted it cut as *Mean Girls* was aimed at a PG13 audience. Almost the same time, the PG13 *Anchorman* was released, which included a visual gag in which the lead character, Ron Burgundy, has an obvious erection. And not a semi- or even a standard-sized one but what Christina Applegate describes as a 'massive' erection. This scene, however, passed muster. So, no to the wide-set vagina but yes — massive erection! The *Mean Girls* producers pointed out this inherent sexism and their line went through.

I've always wondered if what really offended the censors

wasn't just the word 'vagina' but the idea of a wide-set one? If the character had said, 'Someone said I'm lying about being a virgin because I use super-jumbo tampons on my hoo-hoo,' would the line have passed?

But then it's always been like that. For centuries, women have known little about or been banned from understanding how this part of their body works. They have either whispered tiny bits of fanny information or, like my relatives, spoken in code. Everything to do with 'down there' is spoken of in whispers and shrouded in secrecy and shame. A deeply religious family might not even mention the mechanics of getting your first period, so it arrives like a terrible shock.

We've been afraid to ask questions about what goes into our fannies and/or comes out for fear of being thought rude or sinful. We've been reliably informed that during certain times of the month we are 'unclean'. Over thousands of years, holy men have expressed fear and (usually) downright disgust at our fannies. Only very recently, in 1998, was the full anatomy of the clitoris, that seat of pure pleasure, even discovered (by Australian urologist Helen O'Connell).

Why so late? Hmmm. Could it have *anything* to do with the fact that the clit has no reproductive function and is a primary source of female sexual pleasure?

Millions of women and girls, myself included, have been subjected to FGM to 'control' our sexuality and make us fit for marriage. And yet women and girls, the owners of this body part which inspires such fear, terror, shame and pleasure, have had the least to say and share about it. Women are regularly encouraged to flagellate themselves over demented standards of physical perfection, the current toxic craze being labiaplasty. Perfectly normal vulvas are being sliced and stitched – or 'refreshed and rejuvenated', as the plastic-surgery ads would have us believe – into a 'Barbie Vagina', a term coined by Dr Red Alinsod in 2005. Strangely, I haven't heard of any men requesting a 'Ken'.

This is a book which hopes to redress that imbalance.

I've spent most of the last five years of my life fanny-ing about. I don't mean that I've wasted the last half a decade but that I've worked damn hard to raise awareness of the practice of FGM by talking to politicians, the media – in fact, anyone who will listen – about my other half, aka fanny. I call mine a fanny but there is a whole multicoloured canvas of words for the fanny, some coy, some silly, some very rude indeed. How about:

Foof, fanjo, lady garden, muff, minge, down there, pink hole of Calcutta, twat, vajayjay, pussy, Cupid's warehouse, Minnie, Privy Council (brings new meaning to Elizabeth I calling for her Privy Council), growler, the vortex, vulva, cunt and vagina.

I just prefer 'fanny' when talking in a formal setting. I will talk later in this book about the relationship I have with 'Asha', but for now let's just say my fanny and I have been busy over the last few years.

I can almost feel the heat from your face as you read this. It's not very British to talk about fannies, it's not very polite; in fact, it's downright rude. But more than 50 per cent of the world population has one and it is the one thing that links us wherever we live, whatever our culture; all women have a relationship with their vagina and we all go through key experiences.

In 2011, when I first talked about my experience of FGM, I knew I was one of 140 million women globally who had been cut. But I also knew I was one of billions who had a vagina and, from talking to women, I learned that this amazing hole held so many deep and different stories. I have been known to object, on account of the many incredible stories I have heard, when men are called 'cunts'. The cunt, the female hole, is full of depth and warmth, and that is what many of those people who are called cunts lack.

There is an incredible power in sharing stories. I feel sorry for men sometimes; I mean, it's mostly due to how they are raised and social pressure, but they can work next to someone for forty years and not know where they live. And when they talk about sex it's almost impossible for them to reveal any kind of vulnerability. But within fifteen minutes of meeting each other, women will be discussing what brand of tampon they use. Years ago, when Freud was thundering on about vaginal orgasms, I imagine two women having a whispered conversation:

'I've never had a vaginal orgasm,' says one, and the other woman says, 'Phew – me neither. My husband thinks I'm frigid.' A pause. 'Hmm, maybe he's just really bad in bed? Have you tried stroking that little nub of flesh that won't be fully understood until 1998?' Of course, this is the very quantum leap I take to a situation where I am the one organizing a movement for 'orgasm equality', maybe called 'Oh boy'.

Women have always shared more intimate details than men. One man meeting his girlfriend's friends for the first time admitted to being far more scared than when he met her parents. Why? 'Because her friends know everything.'

This book aims to collect stories of women's experience of being a woman: their first period, their first sexual experience of pleasure, their search for that pleasure, their pregnancies – the reality of it all, as well as everything in between and the menopause. Yes, that final *star-trek* ... Women and girls globally inhabit extremes, from a woman in the White House or a palace to the Syrian refugee in a white tent. Their lives could not be any more different, but when their period comes, when they experience their first orgasm, their first pregnancy, or the menopause, they are, in some way, equal. Maybe unaware, maybe scared, but changed for ever.

We've had the vagina monologues; now it is time to start the vagina dialogues. Sharing stories and experiences with women and girls, having conversations, is what this book is all about. Because when it comes to the fanny there is no such thing as over-sharing. Trust me on that. I have written a whole book about it. I have also seen my openness lead to the tangible reality that by 2030 seventy million girls will be saved from FGM.

1. Periods

'Precisely what menstruation is is not yet
very well known.'
— G. Stanley Hall, psychologist

'Over half the world menstruates at one time
or another, but you'd never know it.
Isn't that strange?'
— Margaret Cho, comedian

Across the world, it's said that, at any given time, 334 million women and girls are on their periods. While that sounds like a scarlet party, the reality is that each and every one has a different experience, from Chelsea Clinton and the Duchess of Sussex to a girl from Central Africa. So, we know there will be differences, but every girl and woman has had a first period. Periods are the great equalizer. It doesn't matter whether you're in the White House or looking through the flaps of a refugee tent, if you start menstruating unexpectedly, it's messy and embarrassing. Period.

In this chapter I will be talking to women from across the world about their first period and what it meant to them. I really wanted to talk about how bloody it was, because we're led to believe it's all about blood, but what I found was how personal it can be. How those first drops change both the women's lives and their world. From the girl in Kenya whose period was the sign of womanhood and therefore the end of innocence to my over-organized friend from Finland whose period came in neat ice cubes. This chapter will investigate that very first period. Because, while we all knew it would come, some of us longed for its arrival while many others dreaded it. Some of us, I know, never got it, and those women and girls are also part of this book, just not this chapter. The arrival of blood and what that means is the basis of this chapter, as it changed my life and many of the women I met along the way.

I can't remember now if it was the summer holidays or a Saturday, but I started my period at home in the afternoon aged fourteen, on a warm day. I remember screaming my head off and thinking, *I am going to die*, even though the woman from The Always Puberty Education Programme had come into our school in Year 8 to tell us all about periods, to explain how we could all be our *most unstoppable self* and, presumably, also dedicated buyers of Always products. In the session, she gave us a pad and a tampon each (were we meant to use both?) and told us to put them in a special pencil case with a pair of knickers for when we started *because you never know when your ovaries are going to surprise you into womanhood*. What she didn't do was illustrate how well the tampon or pad held the mysterious blue liquid we saw on the telly ads. Neither did she explain how we'd probably have an overwhelming compulsion to go waterskiing, skydiving and rollerblading, as we also saw in the telly ads. So I was all prepared. I knew exactly what to do. *All* my period had to do was start at school.

Of course, it started at home. A kind of metaphor for its general intransigence.

If I were fourteen today and starting my period, I'm sure I would give it an Instagram account (*Nimko Ali's Scarlet Valley*, anyone?), but in 1996 I just screamed, 'Mum, I'm dying!' It wasn't painful; it was just the bright scarlet colour that freaked me out. It wasn't red like the red of the EU passport we've lost. That would be too deep, like the pain from Brexit I still feel; it was more a London bus red. Shocking enough to take your breath away but also interesting enough to have a closer look. We've all done that, haven't we? Peered at the tampon or our gruesome underwear. We want to see it, touch it, maybe even have an experimental sniff. It comes out of us, so maybe it's a tad yucky but that also makes it okay. It's part of us.

But instead of reaching for my special pencil case I had to use Mum's mega mattress-pads. Not only did they make me walk like a sumo wrestler, they shifted around in my knickers and rustled like chip paper. That night, I lay in bed feeling achy and pissed off with everyone, but particularly that bloody Always woman. Your *most unstoppable self*, my arse.

I know I keep going on about this, but I felt sort of hoodwinked by my own body. In Year 6 (the last year of primary school), my friend Jamie got her period, or what Miss called 'the Change'. *The Change?!* Wasn't this something I'd heard old women over thirty muttering about? I was even more confused. Our class was then asked to be nice to Jamie and told she would not be doing gym that week. The jammy minx! To my ten-year-old brain, this meant that all I had to do to miss hated gymnastics was to get *the Change*, whatever that was.

Another reason that led me to think that my first period would start at school came in Year 8 as I sat in English class. My best friend, who had never missed a day of school, wasn't at the bus stop as usual that morning. There were no iPhones or Facebook back then, so I had no idea what was going on with her. But as I sat in the English classroom I saw her walk in through the school gates. I was so relieved to see her but I couldn't figure out why she was so late. Lunchtime seemed hours away and, as we read *Of Mice and Men*, I made up a million reasons for her lateness in my head. Had she had a doctor's appointment? No, she would have told me. Had someone died? Unlikely, as she wouldn't have come in at all if that had been the case. Maybe – no, it couldn't be – maybe Jason from Take That had replied to her fan letter and declared his undying love, leaving *me* with the piano player? That was it. I was so wrapped up in this scenario that when the teacher asked me the name of the character who looks after Lennie, I replied, 'Gary Barlow.'

Finally, over lunch she confided that she'd got her first period. I was eager to find out if she'd used her *special pencil case*, but apparently not. She had gone home to get changed and her mum had some pads stored and ready. I didn't see what was so great about starting your period, but I tried to show enthusiasm. 'Did they have wings?' I asked. 'Yeah,' she said, an old hand already, 'but Joanna said I should try tampons next time, as the pads always end up halfway up her back.' I told her not to listen to Joanna, seeing as she gelled her fringe to her face and therefore knew nothing about the complexities of being a woman. (Harsh, but I did not like Joanna, who I refused to call Jo, because we were never going to be cool like that. She was just one of those people who never understood boundaries, not at lunchtime, when she would take stuff off your tray, not in class, when she would ask you silly questions as you focused, and now, it seemed, not when it came to your best mate and giving her advice. I mean, who does that?)

When I started my period, apart from the horror of thinking I was dying, I remember the call my mum made to my grandmother. 'Nimko has started her period!' she yelled down the phone with great pride. My grand-mother only lived around the corner, and so she came running. Before I knew it she was hurrying up the stairs to my room, where I lay on my deathbed like Camille (yeah, I am milking it). Gran wafted in, smelling sweetly of the familiar creams and perfume only she could mix, and kissed my forehead. As she gently smoothed my hair out of my face, I remember feeling at ease and thinking maybe this time I wasn't going to die. That feeling was very short-lived, as the dread of imminent death was replaced with embarrassment. Within what seemed minutes of my grandmother finding out that my ovaries had kicked into action, she was planning a celebration feast. I wasn't sure what exactly we were celebrating, whether it was my 'dying' or the blood leaking via Mum's mattress-pads on to my knickers, but my grandmother had ordered a whole half a lamb and was planning to invite the entire extended family to celebrate my becoming a woman.

I said nothing. Instead, as I did for the next ten years or so when I was on or due, I played the melodramatic bitch. Looking at my family as they ate and talked, it seemed odd we were celebrating (and celebrate we did) but that no one really knew why. My little brothers and sister were just excited to get some fizzy drinks. I was excited about the lamb, but I had no idea why my bleeding was such a cause for extravagant celebration in the first place, as no one apart from my mother and gran knew I had started my periods.

Periods, like FGM, seemed to be an unspoken rite of passage with the women in my family. It was expected, we would all have it, but we would never speak about it openly. In that moment I learned that this bloody thing was something not to be discussed. We all knew, we all accepted it, but no one had the words to talk about it.

As I sat, mattress-pad still rustling, and ate the feast, I noticed a glance pass between my mother and my grandmother. Not until many years later did I realize that it was one of relief – maybe they had thought that, because of the FGM, I might never have a period, or something might go wrong. But now, I'm sure, they assumed I had, in their eyes, become a woman. I stress in *their* eyes, as Britney's 'I'm Not a Girl, Not Yet a Woman' still sums me up fifteen years later.

I'm not sure about you, but since my first period so much has changed. When I started bleeding, the mere idea of a tampon filled me with horror, but a decade and a half later, here I am, boiling a mooncup to ram up my fanny. The mooncup is what we should all be using – it's healthy, cheaper and more environmentally friendly in the long run. But the thing about the mooncup is you must be proper in touch with your fanny; you need to love getting right up there with your fingers and not mind getting blood on them. Think about that time you were drunk and woke up wondering if you took the tampon out before you put another one in? That moment you had a good fumble up there for a stray string? Well, that's the kind of fanny intimacy (fantamacy?) you will need in order to use a mooncup. But here's the most brilliant thing about the mooncup – once it's up your fanny properly you won't feel it, and it forms a seal so there is no leakage, regardless of how heavy your periods are. It really is the super injunction of sanitary products – no leaks ever. There can be, however, a slight splatter matter if you're having a heavy period and need to change your mooncup in a public toilet. Just make sure you are sitting right down, insert your fingers and ease that mooncup out with a *shclooop*. The blood in the mooncup will splash round the inside of the toilet bowl, so don't stand up suddenly. When you glance down you'll see your hand has gone a bit Lady Macbeth. This is where hand wipes are your saviour.

You will also need to boil the mooncup for a few hours before first using it. This is fun because you then also have the moral dilemma of whether to buy a new pot to cook your mooncup in or not. Or watch guiltily as your partner blithely heats up milk for coffee in the same pot you use to boil your mooncup <insert terrible joke about a splattiato>.

As I write this, I'm on a flight to Australia, on my period, which these days doesn't seem to last for three days and then just stop, like in those halcyon teenage years when my period was merely a red dribble. My period always rears its bloody head at the worst moments, but by the end it's meant to be a tired dribble of old brown gunge, not a Stephen King *Carrie*-style bloodbath.

I've since learned that female cabin-crew members regularly cope with erratic periods because of the multiple time zones messing up their circadian rhythm. And that an abrupt drop in air pressure when you're on day five can cause a sudden heavy flow, so here I am, asking a member of the cabin crew for a pad.

I'm okay asking for pads, tampons or whatever right now in my life, whereas my teenage self would be dying of embarrassment. My fanny (Asha) and I have nothing to be ashamed of, but what I'm not okay about is that here, on this flight, there was no emergency pad stocked somewhere if they were not in the loos. I looked around three toilets like someone who had lost the phone that was in her back pocket. We all know that crazy search full of panic and the feeling of *It has to be here, it has to be!* Well, that was me when I found myself bleeding like it was day two days after my period was due to finish. When I had given up on finding pads and rejected the idea of using paper towels I asked the perfectly dressed woman at the back of the flight and I was shocked that she had to go into her own bag to get me a pad. She was either also on her period, or waiting for it, so why didn't they just have a supply in the loo? I mean, there must be over forty women on this flight right now on their periods or about to start their period. WTF?!! What are you supposed to do if your period arrives and there isn't a compassionate cabin-crew member on board? Stuff your pants with toilet paper or leak on to the seats, that's what. I would want to do the latter, but that would be cutting off my nose to spite my face, as it would mean sitting there in my blood till I got to Oz. Yup, bleeding down there while travelling down under.

But maybe if a few more women leaked on planes the airlines might have to provide more pads and tampons onboard. The seats might be fire resistant, but I doubt if they're blood resistant too. They say they carry a 'limited supply'. Where? Certainly not in the airline toilet. And why a 'limited supply' when they seem to have an 'unlimited supply' of booze? When you have a period emergency in an airport, it usually means rushing to the nearest tampon vending machine to read the 'Not in Use' sign on it.

Wouldn't it be great if you started your period mid-flight or had the day-five womb gush from the pressure drop and were confident enough to ask for help over the tannoy? 'Ladies and gentlemen, my name is Nimko, and I need a really big . . . tampon.'

My period life has been full of many ups, downs and WTF moments. The WTF moments, like any of us, have been the *why did you not tell me you were coming?* and the most embarrassing of these was just a few months ago when I was on a UK government weekend trip in the country. I was staying in what I would imagine the room of a not so important royal would look like. Full of art and sheets as old as time but still super posh. I had no idea I was due, but maybe due to stress, there it was, all over the expensive and I am sure can-never-be-replaced sheets belonging to Her Majesty's Government. Had this happened even five years ago I would have freaked and tried to hide all evidence of my womanhood, but I did not. I removed the sheets and left them on the floor, and when I came back that afternoon from a high-level meeting I had new sheets. I know the women and maybe even the men at reception knew what had happened – maybe even the British Foreign Secretary knew – but who cared beyond the first WTF of waking up in a bloody sheet.

An up moment was when I worked out that I could get a week off Ramadan while I was on my period. I say a week as, from the moment you start your period, until you wash from head to toe, you would be and are deemed unclean and, as such, you are unable to fast. Of course, I was not on my period for a week when I found this out but what I read in the small print of the Quran was that if, for example, I had nail polish on when I had a purifying wash, it did not count. I stretched it out because it made me feel normal in a world where finding a common ground with those around me was difficult. As a teenager, I really embraced those periods during Ramadan – it meant I could eat with my friends at lunchtime, I could go out to the shop at break and go over to hang with my friends after school. I never felt guilty then, but writing this, I do, and maybe when I bled for ten days non-fucking-stop when I had the coil fitted, I was being punished. I hated my period during those ten days and I was happy to have my ovaries removed and be done with this shit. I wish I could ask someone like Michelle Obama to over-share her period story. Imagine if she had to send the Secret Service out to get her some tampons during a tense meeting in the Situation Room. Her code name was Renaissance, so the Secret Service guy would be in the drugstore on his walkie-talkie: 'Affirmative. Target seen next to the boxes of panty liners. One box of tampons with applicator?' 'Negative – Renaissance wants the ones that expand width-ways to fit you better.' Or if Michelle had the Talk about periods with Sasha or Malia in the Oval Office. I would totally do that; talking periods in the Oval Office – fucking amazing. Me nodding sympathetically while Michelle confides that all that flying on Air Force One messes up her cycle ... Sorry, I was daydreaming.

Currently, women's healthcare is being decided by a group of rich white men, and when I say 'decided', I mean 'destroyed'. These Republican saviours of morality are also vehemently anti-abortion (unless their mistress gets pregnant). Remember that 2017 photo of Trump surrounded by his gurning cronies, all busily proposing to slash women's healthcare? Women make up 51 per cent of the population and there were zero per cent of them in that room.

As we speak, 334 million women are on their period, and some of them have been kind enough to share their first-period stories with me. What's it like to start your period as a refugee, miles from anything familiar? Or, when nobody tells you what a normal period is, how do you know when you have severe endometriosis? How do you cope when your ovaries kick in on a snowy mountain? Or when your bowels go into overdrive along with your ovaries? And how does a homeless woman deal with her period? Most of the time, she has to decide between eating and bleeding.

Zay

'In that dark, cold concrete courtyard, my blood dropped like the tears from my eyes.'

We left Syria three years ago, when I was eleven.

If I had known we would be travelling for so long with nowhere to call home, I would not have chosen my jeans and Hello Kitty jumper as the main things to pack. I loved Hello Kitty, and I still hope someday to go to

Japan and buy as many Hello Kitty things as possible. It's not so much the stuff as what Hello Kitty represents to me – joy, friendship . . . freedom.

We left in the family car with my mother, father and little brother. My mother said we could both take a little bag, and my brother took toys and sweets. We really thought we would only be away for a few weeks. We drove for hours, then we moved on to a bus and then a boat. The boat was the scariest thing until the day I woke up covered in blood. We had been in Greece for two days after weeks of travelling. I had been in pain for days, but I thought it was something I ate or just fear. I prayed every night with my mum, to take the fear and pain away, because she had hurt her back carrying my brother while my father carried me when I could not walk any further.

Then one night I woke up screaming. I thought I had been shot. That was always my fear – people were getting shot in Syria, it was why we left. My mother, who was sleeping next to me, jumped up to see what was going on. She saw the blood, and there was shock on her face, but not horror. Looking back now, I guess she knew what it was. So, she wrapped the sheet we were sleeping under over me and stood me up. We were in a big room, along with other families, and she did not want to attract attention. We rushed out of the room and into the courtyard. I did not say a word – I was just shaking. It was cold, but I think it was the fear that made me shake. There was a tap in the yard where the men washed their feet and got ready to pray. Behind this tap, while holding the sheet up, my mother started to wash away the blood. She wiped me down with the nightdress I was wearing, and as she did she explained that everything was okay, and Allah had chosen that night for me to become a woman. My mother had known this day was coming but hoped it would be when we got to Germany, where we were heading. I was not hurt, she said, it was just my body moving from one stage to another. My mother is a softly spoken woman, and her words always make everything better. But she could not make that better. In that dark, cold concrete courtyard, my blood dropped like the tears from my eyes. My mother was also crying, but I said nothing. It was all so painful in so many ways. We had nothing, I was aching, and she must have felt so hopeless.

She left me for a moment to pop back into the room where we were sleeping and returned with some under-wear and a sanitary towel. The underwear was hers, so she tied it on one side, but there was still space between the pad and my private parts, so there was a lot of leak-age when I went back to sleep. In the morning, I could look for my own knickers, but I had to keep the same pad. My mum had only brought a few sanitary towels with her and there was no way of getting any more. Just like with the rice, milk and bread, we had to be careful with the pads Mum had. I tried to stick to the one a day, but there was a lot of blood and it got uncomfortable. Mum sacrificed herself for me; she was also still having her periods, so she gave me the ones that she needed for herself. I took them like a child, having no idea what I was doing and assuming everything was about me. I took them without a second thought. That might have been one of the last childlike things I did.

Children are selfish, which is fine. They don't know the world is not all about them and, if they have good parents, they *are* told they are the best and it *is* all about them. My mother loved me and my brother. Back home, she would say she loved us every day, and if there were any sweets on the table when I came in from school I would take them and eat them, though after my brother was born maybe I would leave him one ... maybe ... but it was always about me and my brother and *our* needs. When it came to my mum and dad, they left Syria well before the people you see on TV – they left before it got harder. Not that it wasn't hard to travel across borders on your period. My mum said she was crying from the cramps while a baby jumped up and down on her back. I had no concept of cramping and there were no pain-killers. I had no idea of these things and, when my mum told me I was 'becoming a woman', there was no talk about what this meant.

So I had the luxury of pads and Mum had newspaper or one of my brother's shirts. I saw her washing out blood from the cloth one evening, and it was in that moment I realized that she needed the pads I had been taking. I felt yucky, which I always did for days, even after the period had stopped. Not being able to wash as and when you wanted to, not having real toilets, is disgusting, and you feel it. My first period lasted for five days, and at night it would get on my nightdress. My mother cut up a plastic bag she had been using to keep our feet warm when we walked for hours in the rain. I am not sure if it was hours, as it was three years ago, but it was raining. So, the bags were so important for keeping our mattress dry and keeping what little I had in terms of clothes from getting messed up.

I was lucky, as lucky as I could be in my situation, that I only had two periods before we moved to a site in Greece where we could get some aid and support.

The women from the women's centre didn't ask questions like they do when we get food. They just gave us a pack of pads, wipes and some underwear. The underwear was limited, but it was in a box and you just got it if you needed it. It wasn't the same with sugar; they did limit that, and sometimes you didn't even get anything.

My mum feels bad about it all. I overheard her talking to my father before we came to settle here and applied for asylum. She said that I was 'growing up', which I think he understood, if not the line 'She is in pain and I have nothing to give her.' Maybe she should have made that clearer to him. I don't think my father ever understood that periods can be painful and that a mother seeing her child in pain is a terrible thing. Had we gone to Jordan and not come to the West, when my period started, for my own safety, I would have had to get married. It's because unmarried girls can be harassed or attacked at school, so families see marriage as something to protect their daughter and their family honour.

Now, though, I am here, as safe as I can be out of Syria, and I can get a painkiller when that sharp pain hits. I can go to bed in the evening with a hot-water bottle and I can also have pads in my own room and not feel bad or have to ask to use them.

I have wanted to ask my mum about her experience but just did not know how to. It is not what people ask, and it is not even something you think about; it just happens and you get on with it. But when I think about it I remember how hard, life-changing and different it all was, so maybe it is *not* something that just happens.

My mother says she started her period early and it was scary, that no one in the family talked to her about it. Her own mother was too busy having babies and her aunties were married and only spoke to her about the need to address her unruly eyebrows or no one would marry her.

It was finally the older sister of her schoolfriend who told her what a period was and what to do. So my mother planned to be different when she had a daughter, but it was not meant to be, and she said we should not be sad about it all as the Lord sends things our way to test us.

'Tea?'

That is where our conversation ended. I had opened a door into their relationship, which I am sure was always there but was now shaped and located in a different place.

I could only see that as looking at Zay and her mother I saw me and my mother. So far from what we both knew, so young and yet to find a way to express ourselves. I hope my conversation with them about something so personal allows them to see that they really are one and as they grow as they will into these women so different from all those who came before them they find strength in the difference. For me and my mother the unsaid words built walls – even at times if they were just paper thin – they were strong enough to stop us from finding the relationship we have today. A relationship based on love, respect and acceptance of our difference. I will never be the daughter my mother wanted but that is not a failure and today we both accept that. Blood and its role in our lives is deeper than we think. In that room there was so much love, so much unsaid, but so much to come in the next few years, just like the many periods of her life.

From taboo to hang-gliding

I thought that maybe Zay's first period might have been less frightening if her mother had been able to talk to her about it. But speaking in euphemisms, about 'becoming a woman', or just leaving it as a bloody great shock to their daughter, is not uncommon among women, even those who don't have the excuse of fleeing a war-torn country with their baby on their back. The very word 'taboo' comes from the Polynesian word *tapua*, which means both 'sacred' and 'menstruation'. In the West, period taboos seep through our culture in different ways.

In 2016, a fitness centre in Georgia, USA, put up a notice asking women on their periods not to use the pool.

Apparently, chlorine gets rid of sweat and urine, but a few drops of menstrual blood is a bio-hazard? Tampons aimed at young girls are often covered in what resemble sweetie wrappers, presumably to prevent the horror of your peers realizing you have bodily functions.

Adverts are the leveller, and shame is slowly being chipped away. In 2017, Bodyform showed an advert featuring red liquid on a sanitary towel. And, amazingly, the world didn't end. Maybe the next step would be to show women groaning and hugging a hot-water bottle instead of going hang-gliding.

Yasmin

'And I could have ended up being married to someone who would make me live where I had to wash a cloth by the river and live in a village where I had to hide that I was on my period.'

I got married six months after I started my period. I remember that still to this day, even though I now feel differently about my husband and the marriage.

It started on 12 April, a week before my fifteenth birthday. I was in the middle of English class when I felt this need to go to the toilet, but as I knew Ms Lee would give me the stink eye and refuse, I did not bother asking. It was not painful but just like when you are running for the loo and you release a drip or two on the way. When I got to the toilet it was disgusting; there was what looked like a slug in my pants. I really thought it was a baby slug or worm that had come into my pants from somewhere. It was all black, slimy and wet. I almost fell off the toilet looking into my pants.

Because I had to get to the next class and the evil toilet ogre would be coming to check for people bunking off class, I actually flushed my pants away with the dead worm, which I now know were the first blobs of my period. I had no idea at the time, but those few blobs led to a moment in my life that I will never forget. As I pulled up my tights and ran to class, I had no idea that blood was still coming out. As I sat in class waiting for break so I could really have a proper look, drops of blood were still oozing through my tights and on to my skirt. I was not aware of this until I went back to the toilet again at lunch to inspect my tights and I found smaller worm blobs there. Looking back now, it seemed a tad heavy for the first time, and I think I may have started the day before and did not notice and that today, the day I thought was day one, was actually day two. In retrospect, it makes me a bit sad because, without realizing, I missed the momentous moment.

This is how my period was till I had a baby. The first day would be light, just some blood on the loo paper, and the horror show would be on day two, and day three would be 'in bed day', as if my back was breaking. That first time, though, I was not able to leave school, so I made do and used those harsh green only-used-in-prisons-and-schools hand towels as a makeshift pad. This was marginally better than the thin toilet paper there in the loo. It all held up and, when I got home, I ran right to my room to dig out the shoebox where I had put the tampons and pads I was given when I first started high school.

I did not think it was a major issue, so I did not tell my mum until the next morning. I had gone into the bathroom with a small make-up mirror, and I was taking too long, it seemed. My little sister was knocking like crazy and, because she can be a little bitch, she told my mum I was putting on make-up, knowing that my mum would knock down the door at this information, which she almost did. So, Mum basically came flying up the stairs, and I opened the door to inform her and sis that I was *not* putting on make-up but trying to work out how to use a tampon and *that* is why I took my make-up mirror in there.

The look of horror on my mum's face is something I have only seen once before, and that was when my older brother was kicked out of school for smoking weed. I know the idea of me using a tampon, or rather attempting to use one (as I did not have any success), was as bad as my brother not only committing a crime but also getting kicked out of school.

I saw the look, but I rushed past, thinking she was just overwhelmed by me becoming a woman, and got ready for the school bus.

When I got back home from school that afternoon my mother and father were in the kitchen and they called me in as soon as they heard the door. I had always known I would have an arranged marriage, but I thought it was years off. I had no idea that my period would be the trigger. I was in Cardiff, not South Asia, but it seemed that our trip which was planned for that summer would now be used to look for a husband for me. I was shocked and confused, but I did not have the kind of relationship with my parents that would allow me to question what they were talking about. I just said, 'Okay,' and went to my room to sit and feverishly search my books for anything about periods or ovaries or men – just so I could understand what was going on. It seemed like one minute I was a child worrying about exams and toilet ogres and the next I was a woman, with period worms and a husband to find. Later, my mum said, 'Bring that make-up down to me later, it is not good for you.' I knew she meant that she did not want me to use the tampons.

Six periods later, we were in my mum and dad's village in Bangladesh, and the summer heat was worse, now that I would have to use reusable pads. I had never noticed what the women washed in the far side of the river. I never needed to, till now. When I got to my grandmother's house my mum asked one of the girls who was helping her to get me some 'cloth'. She took me by the hand and opened a box containing what looked like old cut-up dresses. She told me, 'Put this in your underwear when you notice it is that time.' I forget what she called it, but it was a word I had never heard of. She then told me where to go and wash it, that we should ensure the men don't see, because that would be horrific and the young boys in the village would never let you forget it.

*

I was going to be in the village for three months, so this cloth might be something I would need, or more like something I might have to fake I needed, if the pads Mum had brought ran out. I was hoping, like the perfume and other things she brought from the UK, she would not lock them away. I found out two weeks after we arrived that she wanted me to act like the other girls, but I could still get access to the pads. I just don't think she wanted me to be different from my cousins.

Being on your period, in the heat, as a teen is (trust me) not the ideal time to be looking for a husband. But I was lucky, as the man who asked for my hand in marriage was someone I knew. He was a neighbour and my mum had asked him to look after me when I was younger and wanted to go swimming or play with other kids in the area. He was only a few years older than me and I can now say that I lucked out.

I am now thirty-five and mother to four beautiful kids, and with the love of my life. When I met my husband I was scared and thought my life was over. I wanted to be back in the UK. I wanted to do my exams. But twenty years later I think it was the best thing to happen to me.

My husband is the type of man who can work both outside and inside the house. So, he goes to work, but when he comes home he takes care of the children too. I know that's how it should be, but it is not common in my culture.

After our first child, because I was then unhappy about

getting married so young, he was there for me. He would look after the baby day and night. He still bathes the kids and dresses them and drives them to school before he goes to work. He got a job as soon as we came back to the UK, and us coming back at all was thanks to him. He saved my life, which you might think I should not be thankful for, but I am. I could have said, 'No,' to him, but I would still have had to get married.

And I could have ended up being married to someone who would make me live where I had to wash a cloth by the river and live in a village where I had to hide that I was on my period.

In the last few years we have been able to set up a business and I have been to Dubai, Morocco and other places. And the only thing he asks is when should he book the ticket for me and how much shopping money I need!

He has been patient and always there for me, no matter how crazy and unbearable I've been. He has loved me for *me* and showered me with love and attention. I have never felt less than a queen with him. I learned that, as much as I was forced into the marriage, so was he, but what he chose to do was make it work, and he loved me before I even knew. When you see the pictures of my wedding day, I don't look happy, and I wasn't, but I am now.

Marriage is hard and requires patience. But so does growing up, and that is why, when our daughter started her period several months ago, I thought how young she was, and how young I was when I started. I wouldn't consider my daughter getting married just because she started her period. I want her to continue her education, although I hope that one day she finds a husband as wonderful as mine.

Slouchers and blocked toilets

How should we talk to our daughters about their periods? While you might not want your mum to sit you down with diagrams, a pointer stick and a flow chart (boom boom), being able to ask questions about periods and know that you will get an answer and not an embarrassed silence or worse, anger, is the first step towards breaking down the taboo of secrecy and shame. In a 1958 information film, Molly starts her periods and her mum tells her to stop slouching and sit up straight so her organs 'have room to function better'. And when Molly is invited to go swimming, Mom says no, as she might 'catch a chill' having 'the Curse' and all. Way to go, Mum.

A friend of mine in her late forties says the only advice she received was a sanitary towel shoved under the bathroom door and her mother whispering, 'Don't talk to men.' But another friend who also started her periods in the seventies fondly remembers her widower dad answering all her questions about periods. When she asked him what he remembered most, he said, 'Calling out the plumber twice because you and your sister kept flushing tampons down the toilet.'

Tasia

'I found it is hard being believed, as a woman,
when it comes to your body and the concept
of pain. We are meant to ache in silence,
and that is what I did.'

It was the end of term and I had finally got in with the
cool kids. I was in Year 8 and being born in August meant
I was twelve while everyone else in my year was thirteen,
so it was even cooler that I had got invited to hang with
Victoria. At her house, we jumped into a paddling pool
that, at the time, seemed the size of an Olympic swimming pool. Then I got this odd need to go to the toilet
and I remember running across the grass and putting my
uniform on. I got into the toilet and, when I pulled down
my underwear, there was this brown mark. I was so
shocked and disgusted I had to check the door was
locked. I wiped myself and, as I did not have to poo, I
thought perhaps I had not wiped properly when I had
gone earlier that day. Yes, I was one of those girls who
did a number two at school, so maybe *that* was why I
made it into the cool gang. Not. I went back to the pool,
not thinking much about it again until I got home. I was
getting changed and again there was a brown mark, only
this time it was a jelly-slug-like thing, in my underwear,
and when I wiped, more came off. I ran, horrified, into
my sister's room because I thought I had caught something from that pool; it was not the cleanest place. My

sister was a total bitch to me then. She took a second away from whatever homework she was doing to glance at me and say, 'You started your fucking period, so don't be getting pregnant now.' *Really* helpful. I had no idea what she was talking about and I couldn't talk to my mum, as she was away working. My mum was in the army and so was my dad. They were never away at the same time, as they thought that would be too hard on us.

They have issues – we all do – but for them I guess it makes more sense. War is not something you can leave at the office door. So, I couldn't ask my dad, and Mum wouldn't be calling for another few days. And anyway, those calls were about making *her* feel better and not about whatever issues we had. Dad or Mum or whoever was with us would give us an agenda for the call. I'm not sure if they knew they both did it, but there was really no one we could talk to about our stuff. I just went back into my bedroom and cried. I've no idea why or what I was crying about, but I just did, and eventually I fell asleep. I woke up at close to midnight and just sat there, wondering what I was meant to do. I finally decided to call my auntie in New York. She was the emergency contact we had, and this was definitely an emergency.

I'm so happy I did call, because across the world, over the phone, my auntie talked to me and made me feel so loved and less alone. The next morning, I think maybe my auntie had called Mum, or she developed a heart for a second. I woke up to my sister sitting at the end of my bed, with some pads and a £10 note. 'Take this,' she said. 'I'm not on for another week or so, but make sure you replace them. Take the pack to the shop to remember which ones they are, and get three packs. I keep them behind the loo rolls. I'll make sure there's enough for both of us from now on. Mum leaves me money for this shit.'

I really wanted to hug her, but she would have hit me. Oh, I'm not being fair. My sister really came through for me then, and I loved her for it. We never spoke about it again and we never spoke about periods in my family either, until I was rushed into hospital one Monday lunchtime.

No one tells you what a period is meant to be like and what level of pain is okay. The first period I had was light, brown and over in a matter of two or three days. I don't remember having to change my pads that often. I did change them, but just because I thought I had to, not because I needed to.

It was the next month when it all changed. I woke up in the middle of the night and it was literally as if someone hit me right in the back. Now that I've had a child and know what pain is and isn't 'normal', I can safely say it was even worse than going into labour. I rushed to the toilet because along with this sharp pain came the need to vomit up whatever was in my system. It was Chinese, if you want to know. My brother had come home from boarding school, so we were celebrating, or acting like it, because he was a boy and it was assumed he'd go into the army too. I'm not sure if anyone ever asked him if he wanted to.

The pain was out of this world – astronomical, in other words – and as soon as I stopped puking I sat on the loo to collect myself and have a pee, but before I could really open my eyes and look down, there was this soft *pllp* sound in the bowl. I had not done a poo, so I parted my legs to look. What I saw made me wake the fuck up immediately. I stood up and put my head to the bowl as if I was going to puke again, but instead I stared at this big shiny blood clot at the bottom of the bowl. It was disgusting and yet the most amazing thing I had ever seen. I put my hand into the toilet and tried to pick it up, but then drew it back. I flushed away the clot and went back to bed, stopping off to get a pad from behind the loo rolls.

The clots and pain became regular and I assumed it was the same for everyone. I would wake up in the middle of the night, racked with pain, and I would spend weekends scrubbing blood off my sheets. For years I never thought it was something to complain about. I did like we all did at school, moaning, 'Oh my God, I'm dying,' but that was what we all said. I had no idea my pain was different. I found it is hard being believed, as a woman, when it comes to your body and the concept of pain. We are meant to ache in silence, and that is what I did.

When the shit (or the clot) hit the fan, I was on my way to French on the fourth floor of S block when my legs gave way and I passed out. I had started my period the day before and day two was always the worst. I had taken a million painkillers and wished I could go home, but in the eyes of the school I was not ill. I had tried a few months previously, with no luck.

It seems it was not normal to have blood clots, and it was not normal to be in so much pain either.

*

At the hospital, I should have been diagnosed with endometriosis, but that would mean that my pain would need to be taken seriously. I was young and was told that I would grow out of it. I have no idea what that meant, and all that happened was that I just got better and better at faking that I was okay until I was able to meet a doctor who would listen and send me for the tests I needed. Basically, the pain I had been living with and struggling with was when the endometrial tissue that lines the uterus starts to grow somewhere else, like on the ovaries or the Fallopian tubes. The doctor told me that because it often starts on the first period, you think that's what a normal period looks and feels like. I felt kind of relieved that the awful pain and clots weren't normal, but also angry. If I'd been able to talk about periods, then I would have found out earlier that the pain and clots weren't normal. Maybe 'normal' is not the right word. I am normal – this is who I am and it's normal for me – but it's not okay. 'Not okay' is what I mean, I guess. It is not okay to be in so much pain, and it's not okay that millions of women like me are being dismissed.

No, I'm not 'uncomfortable', I'm 'in pain'

In 2016, John Guillebaud, Professor of Reproductive Health at University College London, said that period cramping can be as 'bad as having a heart attack'. If we could just leave aside for a second the irony of a man confirming something that women have known for centuries, at least it's being acknowledged, sort of. But as Tasia discovered, endometriosis is severely under-diagnosed, partly because, as she said, 'we are meant to ache in silence'. And it's not just young girls from religious families. In March 2018, the All-Party Parliamentary Group on Women's Health said 40 per cent of more than 2,600 women interviewed reported that they had seen a doctor ten times before being diagnosed. Ten times! What's happening during the previous nine appointments? Either women are saying nothing or they're going to the doctor and having their symptoms dismissed or minimized.

We need to speak up more about period pain in general, instead of chugging back the painkillers and struggling on through an opiate haze. In Zambia, for example, women can take a day off a month if they're suffering. Pain may be subjective, but if you're spending a couple of days every month wrapped round a hot-water bottle, unable to function, it is not normal. It's not fucking fair either. If a man came into work, and groaned, 'I'm getting these terrible crushing stomach pains,' would his boss say, 'Oh, just neck a painkiller, you big, whingeing lummox.' I doubt it.

Aime

'It's been fifteen years since my first period and, since then, for four days out of the month, I am on the toilet six times a day to have a shit.'

My periods are disgusting, gross and a big bloody mess – excuse the pun. My ovaries, guts and bowel just explode every month. If it was just for a few days, like normal people, that would be great. But I have polycystic issues. This basically means that, along with all the blood, my already active bowels go into overdrive.

I started my period when I was twelve and, being a good Canadian, I was playing ice hockey at the time. No, I wasn't; I was just hanging about in the yard. I got up from the grass and thought that it was the damp I could feel. So, I headed to the toilet to take a pee. I didn't really need to but just thought I should try, otherwise I might not get a chance later. Maybe I just needed to get away from Aunt Merry and her not so 'merry' ways. Anyway, I remember getting up from going and screaming. I was so shocked. I was the youngest and the only girl.

'I'm bleeding . . . I'm bleeding!' is what I screamed as I tried to work out if I should pull my pants back up and run out the door or just keep sitting and screaming on the toilet. I was sitting there with my legs wide open, looking down at myself with a shocked expression on my face. I wasn't really scared; more confused and just . . . well, grossed out. I'm not very used to wiping much from the front bottom, but now I had to work that out. I managed to calm down in the end, but from that night the sidekick to my period also started.

I've always been regular in terms of my pooping. Three times a day was always my thing. It was a family joke, really. *Aime is on the go again.* They were all jealous, I guess. I had a healthy system; that's what the doctor said. But that night I was woken up with the urge to pass a number two. This is odd as, unless you have the runs, it's not something that you get up in the middle of the night for. I say it's odd, but then I had a poop routine: once in the morning after breakfast, once after school, as I never went into public toilets (oh, the irony) and once in the evening. So the idea of needing to go in the middle of the night was a real WTF moment.

But I got up, went to the toilet and, because I looked as we all do, I was rather impressed to see that I had passed the longest shit I'd ever seen. I was so proud that I told my dad in the morning, just before I went for my morning number two! This time I also had to work out wiping the period blood away, which was brown as well, *and* the number two. I remember someone in the family shouted, 'Don't use too much paper if your shit is really as massive as you say!'

My morning number two wasn't that big, but I used a lot of toilet paper anyway. I needed to make sure both ends were clean. I then went over to the drawer where I knew there were some pads, for my first step into the world as a woman on her period. We didn't have tampons in the house.

My father was freaked out and thought there would be boys and babies now that I had started. I hoped that all I would get would be cramps and blood. That would be funny, only it wasn't, and never has been. It's been fifteen years since my first period and, since then, for four days out of the month, I am on the toilet six times a day to have a shit.

When I was a student it wasn't so bad, but now that I'm working it's just the worst, especially as I'm a nurse. I can't just run off and have ten minutes in the toilet here and there. And it does take ten minutes, as I can't rush it, and when I go I need to ensure it has all come out. I must change my tampon, which I now use. I also have to make sure that, working in a medical setting, my hands are clean.

I can't even keep it in, as it's painful if I try and I would just pass noxious gas, which is not good in a ward full of people (and doctors you have the hots for). I would lose all my credibility. I'm not sure if you have ever met anyone with IBS or gluten intolerance, but it's like that, only just during my period. I've been tested for IBS and tried all the healthy eating in the world, but this is just how my cycle is.

The smell is not as bad as it could be, but what's worse is the need to carry toilet paper as well as wet wipes. I've been caught short several times and I've learned my lesson. There is nothing worse than going into a toilet, sitting down and there being no paper. Yes, I use public toilets now. I got over that years ago – well, I didn't have much choice. Now I always carry tampons, loo roll, wet wipes and hand cleaner in my bag. The wipes come in handy, as rushing means that you can make the mistake of getting the back wiped into the front. I don't want to say you get shit in your vagina, but . . . you can get shit in your vagina, which can lead to a UTI. It's like leaving a tampon in there too long. A blood-soaked tampon is like a Petri dish for bacteria, and women are more prone to UTIs anyway, because our urethras are shorter.

The Jezebel website once posted a story about what happens when you forget about leaving in a tampon, in great sensory detail. 'After ten days it smelled of rotting fish meets sewage meets the Black Death.' So, I'm hot on hygiene.

You can imagine, though, how hard it is to explain my period package to bouncers when I'm walking into a club. I don't know who's more embarrassed – me or them.

Shit happens

If talking about periods openly is hard enough, try discussing your period shits in polite society. It's all down to (surprise!) hormones. After you ovulate, progesterone tends to slow things down, which is why so many women feel bloated just before their period. Advertisers 'help' by showing us a woman with an entirely flat stomach complaining about 'feeling bloated'. Then she eats a sugary yoghurt, we watch a lot of guff about 'digestive transit' and, suddenly, the problem is solved. If only it were that easy. Because bloating can make you feel like your stomach is full of rocks. Then, just as your period starts, prostaglandin kicks in (literally), making your uterus contract. This, in turn, sets the colon into overdrive. To add to this shitshow, if you suffer from IBS it tends to get . . . yep, you guessed it, worse around this time. Aren't periods sexy?

Fosia

'It is kind of expensive, bleeding over 100 per cent cotton T-shirts made in India that are made for memories, not menstruation.'

When I started my period, it was so odd and cold. I was a Somali Swedish girl in the middle of a school skiing trip. No, there was no blood on the snow, but I did think about it. Just imagine it, a splash of scarlet on all those cold, white acres. I really wanted to call Mum and tell her about it, but I knew she would demand I come home right away. This also meant I could not tell my teacher, or my best mate, as she was unable to come.

I had been looking forward to this trip for months. It was my first time away from home and my first time I was able to be me. Telling Mum would also mean she would freak out, even if I was just a few hours away, and she would think I was dying or something – she would for sure be more freaked than I was . . . well, maybe that is not true. I *was* freaked, but I needed to keep calm, as I did not want anyone to know.

I have no idea what expression I was wearing when I came out of the shared bathroom, but I faked some game face to hide my horror from everyone – my teacher, my roommate, even the man who gave me the skis every day – as I walked shakily back to my room.

I was not ashamed or embarrassed, I was just numb to the whole thing. There was no pain, just a mess in my pants. It was not as bad as it is now; there was just some blood which was browner than red. I knew it was my period, as I had been expecting it, and so had my mum. I am the first girl of three, and Mum had a difficult time with her period. Not telling her, I think, could be charity.

I did not have any pads or tampons and I did not want to buy any as, like I said, I was trying to keep it from everyone. So, I used a T-shirt I'd bought from the gift shop for my baby brother. I cut it up and it was kind of like a nappy . . . well, an expensive and branded one. It was not heavy, so I just needed to change it every few hours and the cold, I think, kept it all in there. When I had to change it, I would go outside before lunch or dinner, knowing everyone was in the dining hall, walk through the snow, find a bin as far away as I could and push the used T-shirt pad into it. I think people thought I had started smoking at thirteen or maybe I was seeing a boy. My teacher asked where I was going a few times, but I just made some silly excuse.

I think I only told Mum because I ran out of money and needed some actual gifts to bring back. It is kind of expensive, bleeding over 100 per cent cotton T-shirts made in India that are made for memories, not menstruation. But it was the day before we came back, so it was fine, and there was no chance of her telling me to rush home or her getting my dad to drive through the night and pick me up.

When I did get home, Mum was lovely. I did not get the usual 'celebration' and, being so far from Gran and the rest of the family, I think me becoming a woman in starting my period made Mum miss her own family. She is also one of four girls, she is the middle sister, and I am sure she remembered when her oldest sister started her period and what it was like to have the whole family around. I was the first of her three daughters and she knew that I might be the first in so many ways. She had come to Europe just out of her teens, pregnant with me and knowing only my dad. I don't think she expected me to be walking back into the house having left my childhood behind, without her being with me when it happened. She thought she was still a child and, having not seen her own mum for so long, the idea that now she had a woman at home rocked her world.

I am named after my mum's older sister, the one she looked up to, and I guess that was her way of keeping her older sister with her. I wonder if it was her older sister she called and asked for advice on how to be a mum to a girl . . . or woman. Well, I still don't know what I am. Woman in body, girl in spirit maybe.

Mother Nature is a smirking bitch

What's it like when your daughter starts her period? I don't have children, so I asked a friend. She says that Mother Nature is a smirking bitch, because your daughter's period inevitably clashes with your menopause. It's basically the House on Hormone Hill. She's coping with raging hormones and the fact that the period always starts when she's wearing her best knickers. You're also coping with hormones, only yours are dithering about whether to stay or go, plus, you're dealing with lines, sudden weight gain and stray pubes sprouting out of your face.

When your daughter becomes a woman, it brings up emotional echoes of your own adolescence. My friend added, 'When I started my period, I sent off for a pamphlet called "So Now You're Growing Up" from Dr White's, which featured an illustration of this sanitary belt which resembled some sort of hernia truss. I wanted to ask my mum, but I was too embarrassed. So, I've gone in the opposite direction and probably bore the pants off my poor daughter.'

Em

'He almost had a heart attack when I left my
period pants out. He tried to recover, but let's
just say he could not get it up that night, as hard
as he tried. I would hate to see what he was like
after his wife gave birth.'

I moved to Bosnia from Romania around three years ago, with my brother. He wanted to open a bar and I started working in it when I was sixteen. He had some money, and I have no idea why he chose Sarajevo, but here we are. I started my period late, as I was a gymnast and, till I was fourteen, my body was that of an eleven-year-old, really. I did not eat much and worked out every day – I had this dream of becoming a famous gymnast, or maybe even a dancer. This was not meant to be because, when I was thirteen and walking back from school, I was hit by a drunk driver. They say I am lucky to be alive, but I was seriously injured and had to learn to walk and talk all over again.

I was in hospital for about six months and started my period there. I woke up one morning, and the nurse helped me out of bed. She was walking behind me to the bathroom to help me wash and dress for physical therapy and saw the blood on my pants. I remember we were both confused. I had seen so much blood in the hospital already I didn't recognize it as my period, or even care. She apologized for not checking with me when my period was due so she could give me something to wear and avoid the mess. 'What mess and what period?' was my reaction. The nurse looked *really* confused then. Maybe she thought my head injury had affected my memory. 'The thing that happens once a month,' she said delicately. But I still had no idea what was going on.

Later that afternoon, my mum visited and explained it all to me. I was wearing complicated medical underwear and there was no pain I could point to beyond the fact that I was aching all over, as always. I wish I could say I was excited, scared or even cared. I felt nothing. I just wanted to get out of that damn hospital. But I ended up having four more periods there before I left. They would come when they wanted to, and I would always be as indifferent to them as they seemed to be to me.

I think of my first *real* periods as the ones when I left hospital and was able to care for myself – *they* started in

Sarajevo. When I started living there I had to buy my own feminine products. It wasn't just independence; I was sexually active by seventeen and on the Pill, so I needed to know how to protect myself. I would write down the names of products so I would know which ones to buy again. I have not had issues with my periods, really, but now they seem to be the cycle which my whole life operates around. When I first started dating I met other young Eastern Europeans living here or Americans here for work experience at the embassy. My brother's bar is popular with the internationals and it was a great place to meet men. That is how he sells it now, to the young women in the city, mainly.

I have been married twice now, to rich, globetrotting men, because I always wanted to travel and I couldn't do on my own. My brother would never have allowed it. So far, I have been to NYC and Málaga. I have also had my teeth done, and I was thinking about bigger boobs, but that was too much for my brother and he objected. Because he knows many of the men, I feel safe with the men I meet and am seeing. When I say 'seeing', I mean I just pop down to some hotel room with the man I'm seeing, and we get 'married' by someone who says he's an official, with my brother giving me away. Yeah, I forgot a male relative must give you away, not that anyone has checked he's actually my brother. All this just so we can have sex.

I can't remember the actual day I met my second husband, but I can remember it was five days after my period. This is what I mean about my life revolving around my

47

cycle. Like my ex-husband, he is Muslim and, if I didn't have a period after a divorce, he could not marry me and the sex would be sinful. Sounds fucking stupid, right? It is, but hey – he is wealthy and whatever the fuck makes him feel better – I don't care. So, we had to go through this whole 'marriage' nonsense again. When I say 'married' though, there was no actual wedding, we just went to see a sheikh. Although when I say 'sheikh' – well, that's what he calls himself. Also, I don't think any of these 'rules' are even in the Quran or have anything to do with Islam. But I am not Muslim, and I don't have to be for a Muslim man to marry me, so whatever.

We went to a 'sheikh', like I said, with two witnesses (it's usually the bodyguards or men who work for him). The divorce from his previous wife was just as simple. The man says 'I divorce you' three times, and that is it. That and having to wait for the period, and then the man is officially divorced.

The moral guilt and pressure these men feel about having sex and you being pregnant is odd. They will do right by you; they will feel they are still married to you, until you have the baby. This means you cannot date anyone but they can marry up to four women, even more at times.

I have been read more about periods since all this. My first guy left me abruptly for a family emergency. I later heard that 'his wife was giving birth'. But he left in such a hurry he didn't say, 'I divorce you,' to me. He could have done it over the phone, but he wanted to do it face to face.

What a gentleman. I was fine with it and, anyway, he sent me some money. That is how I got my teeth done. You can also agree payments and gifts ahead of the marriage. I have just said $1,000, which they are happy to pay, but I guess maybe as I get older I might think about it more.

What I read about periods, well, I guess the notion of it being unclean and these men seeing its arrival as a freedom pass from the so-called marriage that protected them from hell – that is interesting. I have never seen periods as unclean, maybe because, when I got mine I had so little control over my body that wetting myself or other accidents seemed normal.

I like that term 'fake husband'. Funny story about my first fake husband. He almost had a heart attack when I left my period pants out. You know, the ones that are still marked by the last time and you only wash them once as you might not wear them out again? This time I did, because he liked the bra and pants set. I had the white bra I wanted to wear with the dress I bought, and its matching knickers were a bit period-stained after washing so – I thought I'd just wear them to the gym from then on. But I wore them on our date, assuming he would take them off in the dark. But oh no, we ended up getting hot and heavy in the lift, so I whisked them off. Then, for some reason, I tried to brush the pants across his face in a sexy way, completely forgetting they were the ones with the bloodstained crotch.

His face! I still don't know if he wanted to pass out or puke. Maybe both. I said nothing. He tried to recover, but let's just say he could not get it up that night, as hard as he tried. I would hate to see what he was like after his wife gave birth. Still, I am sure she lives in one wing of the house and he lives in the other.

Maybe the older I get, the more I will want a man that gets me and loves all of me, but for now this is okay.

'A swarm of bees, if looked upon by her,
will die immediately'

There's a scene in *Sex and the City* where Carrie farts in front of Big. Later, she anxiously explains to Samantha that she's only human. Samantha responds, 'No, honey, you're a woman . . . we aren't supposed to fart, douche, use tampons or have hair in places we shouldn't.'

Men who are revolted by periods are also generally squeamish about women's natural bodies full stop. Everything must be waxed, scented, trimmed and vacuum-packed, with a stamp saying, 'Does Not Sprout Hair or Leak'.

Unfortunately, these views have centuries of religious disgust to back them up. The Bible dedicates multiple verses to how a period makes a woman unclean, *and* anything she touches, as though a period is literally a plague. For Muslim women, fasting for Ramadan while on your period is off limits, as is touching the Quran or stepping into a mosque. One woman tweeted that when caught by her brother eating during Ramadan, rather than just saying she was on her period she said she was 'tempted by food'.

And in the secular world things were just as bad. AD77–9, and Pliny the Elder was one of the earliest period pontificators, writing in his *Natural History* about the effect a period has on a woman: 'Her very look, even, will dim the brightness of mirrors, blunt the edge of steel, and take away the polish from ivory. A swarm of bees, if looked upon by her, will die immediately.' Alas, this view wasn't uncommon in ancient Rome, so nobody laughed at him or told him to fuck off. On the bright side, Pliny died from 'inhaling a noxious vapour'. It could have been Vesuvius, or maybe a woman, dangerously on her period, farted.

The real problem with taboos is that they pre-date language; they are so deeply rooted that even if everyone in the world is telling you that periods are normal, natural and not shameful, it just doesn't sink into your lizard brain. It took centuries to build up the toxic cocktail of fear and disgust that surrounds periods. It's gradually being chipped away, but it's going to take a long time.

Becky

'When men go into the Burger King toilets, they're not stuffing tissue down their pants or looking for an empty paper cup so they can try to wash away the blood that's been running down their legs all day.'

Do you know what's funny? My story in this book could be sold in the bookshop I slept opposite last night. Being homeless in London is so different to Reading, where I was born and raised. I use that term 'raised' loosely. My mother was fourteen when she got pregnant with me and said she tried to keep me but the social wouldn't let her. A part of me still believes that, because it's so painful to think that your own mother didn't want you. Although having met her, I can see why I was taken into care and why, in the end, even they gave up on me. I don't know how to love. My foster family tried but . . . maybe deep down I don't think I deserve love or something.

I was living with a lovely family when I started my period. I had an older foster sister, so when I told her she sorted me out. From then on, my allowance went up and I had money to buy the pads or tampons as I needed. My experience isn't really that usual for kids in foster care. I was lucky, really. Some of the girls I met when I moved into the group home had no one when they started their period, and no money either. They might well have been in the situation I'm in right now.

When I hit my teens I became a nightmare. I wanted to party and drink. I wasn't interested in boys, really, but my mum had popped up and I just couldn't handle it. I started running away. The home I was in would report me to the police and I would rock up when I needed some food or a shower. You're not supposed to get kicked out of a home till you're eighteen. But when I turned sixteen people stopped reporting me missing so I left anyway.

My periods were never painful but, like any woman and especially in the summer, I just needed a familiar bed and a shower that wasn't in some dump and full of people on drugs or on the game. And there was always someone trying it on with you. But under my sleeping bag, on the street, no one knows what or who I am. When you're homeless, you're invisible.

I've been homeless now for a year. My seventh period on the streets is due in a few weeks. Being homeless and on your period isn't something people think about. I'm lucky that this month I have some pads I bought with a pound I found. Pads make more sense, as tampons aren't friendly to hours of sitting and walking. It's also harder to change tampons – where do I find the privacy to do it? And in the conditions I'm living in it would be so easy to get an infection. So, it's pads.

When people think of the challenges of sleeping rough, they think *how do you sleep when it's so loud? Don't you fear you'll be attacked?* Or, *how do you find enough food?* But not about periods. Most of the people on the streets are men because it's easy as women to fall into prostitution or get pregnant so social services take you in. Because of this, a lot of people ignore the gender difference on the streets. When men go into the Burger King toilets, they're not stuffing tissue down their pants or looking for an empty paper cup so they can try to wash away the blood that's been running down their legs all day and then having to scrub them dry. Have you ever tried to dry your legs on one of those hand-dryers? Men don't know the fear of finally having enough money to buy something to eat but worrying about dripping blood on the floor while you wait in line for a bag of chips. That you might be told to leave a supermarket because you stood so long looking at the discount counter that the tissue you had as a pad has fallen out of your pants and is lying crumpled and bloody on the pristine floor. You don't notice it, or the looks from the other shoppers or the security guard, because now you're so busy counting your coins to see if you can afford a drink with the about-to-go-off half-chicken that it takes a minute to notice you're being poked with a pen because the security guard is too disgusted to actually touch you.

Unlike my first period, which I can only remember happened, *that* day, the day of my worst period experience, I'll remember for ever. I hadn't eaten really for a few days, I was bloated and didn't feel that hungry. I wanted tea, just for the sugar to keep my strength up. It was March, so winter had passed but it was still cold. Period blood, being like any liquid, means that when it's cold it doesn't drip as much, and I'd stocked up well that afternoon and had a few napkins in my underwear. When you look like I do, you're always self-conscious. People think you're a drug addict, or a shoplifter . . . the usual. Every second or so I would look up to show I was looking at the food, not for a way to nick it. I wasn't shaking from drugs. I was fine on my feet. As I bent down, it seems the napkin in my underwear had come loose. Honest to God, I didn't feel it rolling down. I wish I could laugh about it now, but I still can't. I was too busy trying not to look like a criminal. I hadn't noticed my greatest fear coming true. Under the bright lights of the supermarket, it fell on to the gleaming floor, bloody and unforgiving.

Before I could show the security guard the money I had in my hand and tell him I was paying for the food I picked up, he pointed to the floor. And then he just poked me with a pen. He was standing as far away from me as he could. 'Get out of here!' he shouted. 'People are shopping for food, for God's sake!' If there was a god – in that moment, I wanted him to take me.

I wanted to run, but I thought the rest of the napkins in my pants would fall out as well, so I walked out of the supermarket as fast as I could, squeezing my thighs together. I ended up spending my food money on a hostel, where I sat and cried. But there I met Mary and, after I'd showered, she came and found me. She saw I was upset and I told her what had happened. Mary put her arms around me and told me about how she'd woken up in a hostel over Christmas and discovered she'd leaked all over the bed. It was ten years ago – she was only seventeen then – and she was terrified she'd be kicked out, so she spent hours hand-washing the sheets and scrubbing the bed. She said that experience had taught her the importance of always having a pad and, if not, to go beyond the loo paper.

As we sat in the middle of this hostel's feeding room she showed me how she made a pad out of cardboard, a plastic bag and some of that paper you get to dry your hands. What you do is cut the shape out of the cardboard, place the paper over it and, as you're unlikely to find tape, you can use the plastic bag on the edges. You can also use the plastic bag as protection between the cardboard and your knickers when it's wet, or if you are having a heavy one.

This is what I use now, when I don't have the money for pads. It's still unpleasant, but it's the only luxury I have.

The 'luxury' of sanitary products

It's bloody incredible that sanitary products are still seen as luxury items. And on top of that, we pay a 5 per cent tax for what the government defines as a 'non-essential luxury item'. So, here's a list of some of the things considered more essential than towels and tampons, all taxed at zero per cent.

- Bingo
- Jaffa Cakes
- Kangaroo meat
- Herbal tea
- Chickpeas

A recent pilot scheme in Scotland to distribute free sanitary products in schools and to low-income families found that, out of 2,000 women, 70 per cent had been forced to use toilet paper in place of a sanitary towel. Sadly, such a scheme is unlikely to happen in the rest of the UK. And despite a few newspapers loftily saying that 'most women' can afford sanitary products in the UK, 138,000 girls miss school every day in the UK because they, or rather their 'most women' mothers, can't afford sanitary protection. And there are countless more, stuffing toilet paper or socks down their pants. The double whammy of poverty and period shame.

2. Orgasms

'So not only was I wanking as often as a boy,
I was also being unfaithful to Richard Gere.
So much for FGM "curbing" me.'

Not all of us have had sex, but we are products of it and it is used to sell us everything from loo paper to cars. Some of us think sex is a right, a human necessity; others have decided it is a sin they can live without. In this chapter, I will be talking to women and girls about the pleasure beyond the act. I will be looking into the role female pleasure plays in different cultures and how some of the myths around female sexuality affect the role of female orgasms. From religion and legislation to the media, the female body is forever under discussion, women and girls are talked about and talked at, but in this chapter I will talk to women about their most powerful experiences and their relationships with their first orgasm, about the pain, the pleasure and pure lust. We talk about our first time, but never the first moment of pleasure. The moment the world made sense for many, that moment when you realize how much power you hold. An orgasm should be like an earthquake. The world should move and, sometimes, it's just what you need to fix all that is wrong. The fact that we talk about and romanticize the first time we had sex – the location, the man – but never get beyond the act is just mad. We are never told to seek equality in orgasms or that we should be counting them and not calories.

I have lived and still live in a world where female pleasure is seen as a bonus, and not the aim of sex. Women are the object when it comes to sex and never the subject. We are there to be fucked and never to be just pleasured.

Pleasure is something I regained for myself. I worked hard for it, and I now guard it and I won't be with a man who doesn't give me pleasure. I'm not willing to sacrifice that for anyone, and I shouldn't feel ashamed about it.

I can't put a finger on my first orgasm, but I do know I had a hand in it. (Sorry about that.) But it is true that, for me, pleasure, and the idea that FGM, which I had when I was seven years old, had taken away a part of me which was meant entirely for pleasure, is something I just could not get out of my head.

When I first started exploring my body, I didn't really know what was possible, but I understood that getting to know myself for pleasure was an act of rebellion. Something had been taken away from me. What was it? Why did it need to be removed and why was everyone so scared to talk about it? In a search for these answers, I found the power of pleasure in myself. I somehow reclaimed it without really looking forward to it and, since then, I have protected it with every part of my being. Ironically, I'd have had far less interest in my vagina had I not been cut. I was curious as to why adults were so interested in my vagina that they cut a part of it away.

If FGM was meant to diminish my desire, it failed spectacularly. It's made me more sexually adventurous, more bold, and you could say brave. I was no longer just interested in what was there and what had been taken away but also why there was so much angry discussion about this folded, hidden part of the female body. What was so special about this hole? Yes, the deep and wonderful hole, but to a teenage me and, sadly, today to millions of women, it was just a hole.

Growing up, I would listen to the women around me talk about sex. Yes, Somali women talk about sex, and they actually talked about it a lot, but they used a sort of schoolgirl code (more later) and never once discussed orgasms or masturbation. I'm sure as I sat there silently, having my hair done and listening acutely, they thought I didn't understand what they were talking about. Or maybe they thought I'd be scared by the fact that they never spoke about pleasure in sex. At all.

When the women in my family and their friends got together, they spoke in Somali, and I knew the word for sex (*wass*), or rather for 'fuck'. In their world you went to bed or fucked when it came to your relationship with your husband, and that was the only context sex ever took place in – in a marriage. When you're a kid, you need to know the key words, and 'fuck' was one of them so, in this context, after a wedding, when 'fuck' was being used, I could only conclude that they were fucking, not being fucked or told to fuck off.

I would listen to these conversations and soon picked up the schoolgirl code; the main thing was that sex was always referred to as 'the wedding night' when it came to the first time, and was, from then on, all the same. Even for the aunties, who had been married for years, the act of sex, or fucking, or getting it on with your husband of twenty years, was always *the wedding night*. So I would listen to my relatives and assume that sex was a marital contract, that it was done in the proper place and always with a man.

Travelling back to my birthplace of Somaliland to hear stories from women there, and trying to explain what this chapter was about, I found that, in my language, there was no word for what we call or know as an orgasm. In Somaliland, a deeply conservative culture, the idea of sexual pleasure was very male (surprise), and even then it was about them 'cumming', a word that literally means 'releasing water'. That summed up what the male orgasm was. I had to sit, and educate women and break down what this chapter would be about. It was not the act but the feeling, the self, the moment. I spent hours talking and listening, this time without the use of schoolgirl code and as an adult, to women who could easily have been my mother, or my aunties, about the notion of sex for pleasure; the idea of a man or those they loved being more than someone to be married to and instead a partner with whom you shared your life.

But as I travelled around the world, women and girls being so taken aback by the idea of openness about sex and pleasure wasn't just something I found in Africa. It was the same in so many other places, from Ethiopia to East London. Maybe me asking stopped them in their tracks. There I was, a Somali, African, Muslim woman who had had FGM talking about pleasurable sex. Over and over I was asked, how could I even know such pleasure? The women and girls I met who looked at me as a Somali and a Muslim couldn't believe it, because they believed that sexual pleasure for women was something that was not in our culture.

But this isn't and never has been true! If they had been allowed or had been able to read the texts of the faith they wore so openly, they would know it was there. Sexual pleasure for women is a central tenet in Islam.

Islam's instructions for husbands from the Quran state, 'Do not begin intercourse until she has experienced desire, like the desire you experience, lest you fulfil your desires before she does' (Al Mughni, 8:136).

Growing up, I'd discovered intense pleasure through masturbation, which took me beyond the boredom of my bedroom. Being older, I could now ask questions. I could contextualize the difference between the act of sex and the experience of pleasure.

The main reason for these questions is that I've been raised in two different cultures. In the first, women basically orgasm at the sight of a topless man drinking Diet Coke, and in the second, I grew up listening to my female relatives talk about sex using a coy code while I rolled my eyes and wondered what they would think if they opened – or, even worse, actually read – *More*, aptly named as that woman's weekly mag was: it was where I got 'more' – in fact, 'most', of my – information about sex. I was a late starter and very keen to catch up, particularly as the wider UK community was my main culture. I was educated and socialized outside my home with non-Somali people.

I was confused. I was also very on edge. My teens coincided with *The Girlie Show*, a Channel 4 late-night 'yoof' programme screened to coincide with the rise of ladette culture. I was glued to it. The all-female presenters brandishing whips! Mounting rocking horses while winking sexily at the viewer! Going to Amsterdam and trying to pick up women in gay clubs! And the highlight of the show, Wanker of the Week. 'What a wanker!' Sara Cox would chortle, waving her clenched fist about to denote said male celebrity's wankerness. On *The Girlie Show* sex wasn't just talked about openly but shoved in your face like a custard pie. Or the money shot. It's since been criticized for blaring out the kinds of stereotypes it was supposed to be reacting against, but I didn't care. It was the first programme where I heard the word 'clit'. And the first time I realized I might be missing something important.

The first flutter of my fanny sent me on my initial journey, but I didn't know that 80 per cent of the clitoris is internal. Nor did I know that my female relatives, who I judged so harshly, actually had no word for pleasure. I had projected my very Western TV shows and reading, which all talked as if people were orgasming all over the place, on to them. I've discussed orgasms and pleasure a lot with women from different cultures, but the main question I get asked when discussing the idea of pleasure after FGM is 'How can you talk about pleasure when you were cut?' This is an interesting question, so before we hear from the women and girls whose first orgasm was with their first, or with their tenth, aged forty, or never, or even with their one and only lover – let me show you, or over-share, mine:

My sexual journey and education began when I was fourteen and reading my beloved *More* magazine. I'd be paying attention to their Position of the Week. Many of these so-called positions made my eyes water and often I had to turn the page upside down to work out which body part was going where. To avoid censorship, they used Ken and Barbie dolls. One position coincided with 'National Stop Snoring Week'. (How to keep your man up all night!) How was that a result? Anyway, Barbie lay on her back wearing black lingerie while Ken crouched between her bent legs. 'Sex-Somnia', it was called. Another feature was 'Recipe of the Week', although it had no relation to cooking – it merely took place in the kitchen. Poor Barbie was balanced precariously in an advanced yoga headstand while Ken merely stood between her splayed legs – presumably wondering where his dinner was. I hate to think.

Besides poring (porning) over magazines, I also watched too much TV that I may have been too young for. Channel 4 in the nineties was somewhat porny to me, with *Eurotrash*, *The Word* and, if I stayed up really late, the Australian cult classic *Prisoner: Cell Block H*, about a women's prison packed full of women who turned to each other in the absence of men, and some who were lesbians. I wasn't bothered by the way the walls in this prison seemed to wobble, or that practically every week they had a riot which consisted of three women running along a cardboard corridor. I was too busy wondering what they did with each other when they closed the door. There was one majorly evil guard called Joan 'The Freak' Ferguson who would sexually harass the women. She may have even raped one. I can say 'rape' – now that, at the age of thirty-five, I know what consent is.

But it was *Queer as Folk*, about gay men in Manchester, that totally shocked me, as I had very little idea about men having sex. It was the first time, I think, that gay men had been shown on television as non-camp. Before then, we'd had men like Larry Grayson and John Inman – gay, but non-threatening and sexless. There was no way the men in *Queer as Folk* weren't having lots of sex.

Being straight and a kid, I had no real idea that what I was watching wasn't the kind of sex I'd choose to have. But being a kid, I was also shocked at how explicit it was. There was no way I'd let any relative of mine watch it. Or any teen. Apart from me, of course. Being more high-brow now, I get that *Queer as Folk* was a groundbreaking coming-of-age drama, but at the time I had a thing for Richard Gere, and the main guy (Aidan Gillen) looked just like him. I just loved *Pretty Woman*. I thought that a rich man buying Julia Roberts for $3,000 was a love story. I could quote every word, and it was where my thing for older men started. Again I had no idea about consent and the power dynamic at play in *Pretty Woman*, but you could say this passion saved me from getting into major trouble because, apart from the fact that I was fat (and I mean massive) till I was fourteen or fifteen, wanting only to fuck older white men called Richard Gere who lived in Los Angeles meant that I was not getting any action any time soon. Sex was everywhere in TV and films, and this was the basis for how half of me thought about sex from a young age.

Back to my orgasms. I don't remember when I first started to masturbate. It just happened. But I did it a lot, and still do. If I'd been a boy, I think my little man would have fallen off. Ironically, growing up, I had no idea that FGM was meant to curb my sexual needs or desires. It would also be fucking odd for someone to say, 'We cut your clitoris and stitched you up so you would not be wanking over Jason from Take That.' Jason was my favourite, way above Richard Gere, when I realized he was too far away for me to run into. Also, Jason looked like Lee, my crush, on that second day in Year 8. (I liked to keep my wank-bank stories as realistic as possible.) So yeah, not only was I wanking as often as a boy, I was also being unfaithful to Richard Gere. So much for FGM 'curbing' me.

Jason was soon relegated to second place when Michael Owen started playing football for England. I spent hours in my room, daydreaming about being a WAG and wearing nothing but his shirt. Honestly, I still can't see him on television without cringing and *What the hell was I thinking?* washing over me. My wank bank has been upgraded since I was fourteen, and you are more likely to find a Tory minister in there than a football player. I won't name any names, but the tall, awkward-looking ones are my faves. I also think anyone that rigidly uptight in public must be a freak in bed. I mean, for God's sake, they must let that rigidity out some way and, in my head, they let it *all* out, for sure. Either that, or they use that rigidity to keep them upright in the saddle when they're out hunting foxes (the four-legged ones).

I started to get what I call *the tingle* down there around the age of fourteen or fifteen. Yes, I was late, and maybe that had to do with my FGM. In fact, I had aches and pains in my back and my fanny till I was eleven, when I had a deinfibulation that basically undid some of the FGM. At first, I didn't think about it again and assumed things would be like all the other girls' now.

After the deinfibulation, I really wanted to get to know my body, my pleasure points. This all started with naming my fanny. Yes, that's right, at fourteen I decided to reclaim Asha from all the bullshit and get to know her for myself. This was a powerful act and it allowed me not to identify my body with FGM. But the older I got, and when I finally started having sex, I realized that in seeing my fanny as something that wasn't connected to me and my emotional needs I was denying myself a powerful emotional bond. The idea that an orgasm could be both physical and emotional is something that, in these last few years, I have learned to accept and embrace. You could say I have not just grown up but also grown into myself.

This chapter will ask women about that moment of orgasm, about the search for it or the understanding of it. I could have talked about and asked women about their 'first' time. Most of us can remember that, but we're talking about orgasms here, and they can be solo, in a twosome or, for some exciting people, even more. Many women, when they masturbate, are more relaxed and focus just on their fanny rather than their partner, so their orgasm is also more relaxed and leisurely – like a warm, blissful wave (or several!) spreading outwards and upwards. I'm not saying sex with a partner can't also be amazing, but part of the excitement comes from their response as well as yours. Sometimes, as Miranda from *Sex and the City* says, 'It's like a race for an orgasm.'

I wanted to make this chapter about the first time we get that feeling – not just the first time we have penetrative sex but about the first time we explore down there. Some feel a sharp jolt, like the moment after we sneeze, some the dizzy light-headedness of getting out of a too-hot bath, or that little blackout we get after drinking too much (*la petite mort*, the French call it), but I'm sure when you really think about it, you'll remember the first time. I am also interested in life beyond the social and cultural idea of sex being something done to women and looked at through the prism of the 'madonna/whore complex'.

Muna

'I was not sad we had done it or even that it hurt. I was really scared that it would all change between us. But in fact, we grew closer and that is when the pleasure started.'

Sex and pleasure have always been important to me and after my rape that did not change. My first time is a before and after that act. I am not sure if many other women feel the same, but for me it was about regaining my confidence and control over my life in every way, especially with taking pleasure in sex. The act of rape is not about sex as much as the organs used, which, in my case, were sexual ones. It was about power and he, the man who raped me, hated me. He hated everything about me and I am sure he got pleasure from seeing me in pain.

The man/boy who gave me my first orgasm was my first boyfriend. I loved him, and I still do. I won't lie and there is no shame in saying that I was hooked on him from day one. That has been my way since I can remember and that is what drove the hate that came at me when I was raped. It was not wanting him that made him think he could take it.

I met my first boyfriend on the bus coming home from school. We were on Acton High Street, it was summer and my skirt was rolled up. I had just learned to shave my legs without a million cuts, so they were out, and I was looking fly as fuck. He was sitting at the back with some other boys and we locked eyes. I had never seen him on the bus before. Seems he was new to the area.

He was hot, and he knew it. I also knew I wanted him when I deliberately stayed on past my stop. We got further and further away, and I was hoping he would get off soon, but it seems he was doing the same thing and we ended up being the last two on the bus. I knew then that I really liked him as I started getting hot and embarrassed, but we waited till the bus got to the station before either of us said something. I asked him if he was from Edgware – there was no other reason for him to be on the bus this far. 'No,' he said, 'but I missed my stop. I was busy with my phone and forgot to jump off.' I knew he was lying about that. Then I told him I was going to see my auntie. Neither of us wanted to admit we stayed on the bus because we liked each other. Although I know he would lie to this day that he wasn't into me. He was. He spoke with a strong accent, which to me was the cutest thing about him.

He was from Hammersmith and I was from Acton. We were only a few stops away from each other. He was from Poland. His family had come to join his dad and brother, who had been here for a few years. His brother was so lovely – we could always count on him. He would let us just sit for hours in his car, kissing, as neither of us could drive but it was the only place we could be alone.

The flyover looking down on us would become the soundtrack of our happiest times. My boyfriend was lovely and, while there was never any pleasure from him, after a year of dating and me finally being open to some fingering, that felt good. I was freaked out by the idea of going anywhere near his 'big man', as he liked to call it. He only said that once and because I laughed so hard he never said it again.

I guess it was not fair that I was having all the fun. It was all touch and go, really (he would touch, and I would go). There was nothing to call an orgasm with that finger play and I think we did it just to make it feel like we were doing *something*. I hoped if he told people that I had let him do that they would stop talking. It sounds bad, I know, and plays a lot into the bullshit I had to deal with, but peer pressure is everything and he was everything to me. I was gripped by it, but because he loved me, and I had no idea how much at the time, but it was because of that that we made it above all the white noise of 'just do it'.

Don't get me wrong. I was grateful that he cared enough to make it special. So many others just did it in a car or at a party somewhere. He knew that was not how I wanted it and he knew how much I loved him too. His brother also knew and gave him some money for a hotel. We lied to our families – well, I did, anyway. Although I am sure he just told his he was going to his mate's house for the weekend.

Looking back, it seems a lifetime ago, and we were so young. We booked a Holiday Inn near Heathrow, so the traffic of the flyover was replaced with flight noise. I got there after him and when I got into the room he had already run me a bath. He'd bought Radox bubble bath – don't laugh – he thought *I* needed to relax, but I think it was him who should have taken the bath. And I did need a bath afterwards, it was so bad and painful. At first it was, like, a little sharp, but that soon passed. After that it was just uncomfortable. It did not take long and when he finished I just wanted to cry. I was not sad we had done it or even that it hurt. I was really scared that it would all change between us. But, in fact, we grew closer and that is when the pleasure started. Caring for him meant that I relaxed when we got into bed together and then it was not painful any more. Nothing makes you less relaxed than someone telling you to relax and to go with it. *Go with it* – such a terrible phrase, it is the worst. The thing is, I have a very small vaginal opening. This is something I only found out after the rape, because I tore so badly. But it was also what made sex so painful for a long time, so pleasure for me became inter-linked with emotional intimacy.

The night my boyfriend and I made love and I finally came was just after my sixteenth birthday. We had sex twice after our first time, and it was painful both times. He knew, as I tried to hide it but I could not. It was New Year's Eve and we were at a house party. As the only couple, we got the bedroom, so it would have been rude, lol, not to have given it a go. But the night when it really happened at last was a spring evening. We had just come back from the movies and we kissed just under the stairs to his flat and I melted into his arms, as I did for the first time. I could feel myself loosening up. That was the first time I could also feel something wet between my legs as he led me to his room. My thighs started to heat up. I was hot for him and, as we walked into his room, I was ready. His room was so small, I have no idea how all six feet of him fitted in there or how we both fitted, but we did and so did our parts that night. The smell of Lynx aftershave was overwhelming, but it was also his smell and on him it was different. To this day, when I walk past excited teenagers or students, the smell reminds me of him. I was loose and relaxed, so my vaginal opening could also loosen up, expand and allow him in. It was beautiful, even if it was a little painful. His kisses and the flickering heat from the candles that almost burned the place down were everything. My orgasm came just as he did; it was the focus that came from deep down – it was like the relief you feel when you rush to the loo just as you are about to wet yourself. I did not wet myself, but I was wet, and he could feel it. We lay there for an hour or so, on this wet spot, both of us too overwhelmed to move. There was no need to move; we couldn't move. But in the morning when we heard his mum coming in from her night shift we moved fast, for sure.

We are still friends, but I moved away for uni and we got busy, so busy that I thought of replacing the friendship we shared for a mutual friend. I had gone to college with the man who would end up raping me and we found ourselves in the same uni town. Birmingham is a big city and, when you are new to town, seeing someone you know is one of the best things. I was so happy to see him, and I thought he could fill the gap of what I was missing. We started to hang out and, as he knew Anwer, my old boyfriend, I talked openly about him. Sex was all we talked about when at school and college, so I saw nothing wrong in telling him everything. I had only been with Anwer and it was true love, but this man joked that I needed to try out other people and see what I was missing.

The night it happened we had all been drinking. I was pissed, but I knew I had no interest in him, and he knew as well. It was so painful, and I cried all the way through. He could not have found real human pleasure in that and, if he did, then he is not human, he is something else.

When it was over he left me there on the bed, weeping and bleeding. There I was again after sex in a wet patch, but this time it was blood and his semen. It took me three days before I could pull myself together and get to the doctor. Have you ever cut the side of your mouth? That sharp, right-to-your-core pain whenever you move it to speak? Ever felt that? That was the pain I felt when I walked to the doctor. I had to, because I had no money for a taxi. I did not report the rape, and I don't think about it much, but it has shaped my life.

It was three and a half years before I got close enough to anyone else to even think about sex, and it was nine months into that relationship that I had my first orgasm. We were on the sofa, after dinner, just reading. He was rubbing my feet – and *boom!*

Footgasm

To describe Muna as 'lucky' is the wrong word after all she went through, but being able to orgasm through her feet does seem like a gift. And how amazing! To be more specific, in the acupressure world, the area between the ankle bones and the Achilles heel corresponds to the vagina. Also, licking and sucking the toes are enough to make some women cum. I'd love to try this one at home and report back, but I'm a few advanced yoga classes away from being able to stick my feet in my mouth. Imagine if women could have amazing orgasms from just sucking their own toes? We could have our own joke: Why do women suck their toes? Because they can.

Laura

> 'How could I say I was rejected for something
> I had no control over?'

He is beautiful, but I have not met him. We speak seven times a day and I long for him. I really do – the way he talks to me and the fact he says he loves me is what keeps me from finding someone here, which would, of course, be easier. We are not going to get married without meeting – I am not that crazy, but maybe you are right. I might be too horny to think straight.

He will be my first, and that is how it should be, but he

lives in Europe, so I have no idea if I will be his first. I really hope so, because the idea of him seeing other women who have not been cut is playing on my mind. I am very insecure about my down below, it makes me uncomfortable, insecure, and it feels like I might not be whole, which I am not, but I am not sure how to get over it.

I am better than I was a few years ago, then it really affected me inside and out. I would spend hours online thinking about what I have and don't have. I would look at pictures of women who have not had FGM, wonder how my body would have developed had it not been cut when I was so young. The pain of FGM for me has not really been physical, it is emotional and mental. I may have not been with someone before, but I have been in love and I have been close to getting married before. When I was nineteen I met someone here in London, he was smart, funny and we really got along. We 'dated' – I use that word loosely, we went to Nando's, to the movies and held hands. Just before he went off to university we decided to get engaged. I was over the moon. He was all I had dreamed of, and he loved me as much as I loved him – well, that is what I thought.

Just before the engagement my mum came to me and asked what our plans were. I had no idea what she was talking about at first, but she was soon clear. I had type 3 FGM, meaning I was stitched up and that I needed to seek medical help if, after our engagement, we wanted to sleep together.

The embarrassment of my mother talking to me about sex was overwhelmed by the confusion and fear of what might be about to happen. Having never hidden any of my fears from Ahmed, I called him and, over a coffee, I told him what my mum had said and asked for his advice. What I got was questions and not advice. I had assumed that because he was also Somali he knew about FGM and that his sisters or mother for sure had been cut. It seems I was wrong, and we left the coffee shop in silence after an hour. He would normally call to see if I got home, but that evening nothing, and it was the same the next day. I tried to tell my mum, but the words were not there. She would have also been pissed off at me for talking to him – a man – about such a thing.

He finally called after days of ignoring my calls, texts and Facebook messages. I knew as soon as I heard his voice that something was up. He tried to brush off the issue of the FGM and said that maybe we should just rethink getting married and maybe we were too young. I was not having any of it and I told him that we were younger when he asked me, and he was excited just days ago. He finally admitted it, and it broke me – he told me he wanted to be with someone who would not have issues. It seemed he had been googling FGM and concluded that, in his words, he wanted someone 'he could have sex with and could enjoy it'.

The idea that sex was beyond the love I thought we had for each other was something that shocked me and rocked my world. I could not tell my mum why we broke up; I had no idea how to, and keeping it all to myself took its toll. I had a breakdown and spent four months in hospital. In there, again, it was odd. As much as I was told to express myself, I could not. How could I say I was rejected for something I had no control over? How could I say, in seeking support, I found rejection?

After my time in hospital I came out and found women who had also been subjected to FGM and I was then able to talk about it. I visited a clinic, where I was reopened, but this meant I now could see what was behind the stitches. I spent time looking at real, uncut vaginas online, and it looked nothing like those. That is the image I have in my head. I have thought about going to France, where there is a doctor who does some reconstructive surgery, but I am not sure about that. They might leave me worse than I am now, or maybe I should just accept myself how I am.

I am no longer worried about what having sex will be like. Not being rejected and being someone who 'he' can make a life with is all I wish for.

My new relationship is different. I have told him, and I was honest about why my last relationship ended, and he has been so supportive. I don't want to say I am surprised, because we have not met and maybe it was just my ex who had the issue, but I feel hopeful.

We met on a Facebook page and after a few exchanges on there he added me as a friend and I accepted. We just spoke about general stuff at first – school, work, family and hobbies. Soon we were messaging daily and when he asked how my day was I found myself telling him. We talked about the odd man I met on the Tube, how I did not get a lunch break and how I was single but did not want to be. It did come as easy and randomly as that, which is why I am hopeful but, then again . . . who knows?

Type 3 FGM

There are three types of FGM and type 3, the one that Laura had, is the most extreme. Daughters of Eve describes it as the 'narrowing of the vaginal opening through the creation of a covering seal. The seal is formed by cutting and sewing over the outer labia, with or without removal of the clitoris or inner labia.'

Not only is this extremely painful and, to be clear, entirely medically unnecessary, it can also cause catastrophic ongoing problems. Because the vagina and the urethra are closed over, leaving only a tiny hole through which to pass urine and menstrual fluid, there is a major risk of infection, abscesses and agonizing labour. Laura was then dumped by the boy she loved. Oh, the horrible irony. Cut to ensure she would be 'ready' for marriage and then rejected because she wouldn't be able to enjoy sex.

There seems to be a major disconnect going on here. Girls are cut because of strong, deeply rooted beliefs about FGM being a rite of passage and a condition of marriage. Parents believe they are doing the right thing. Words like 'decency' and 'morality' are used. It's as though, without FGM, parents really believe that a girl's libido will run wild. But even if you put aside the ongoing pain and mental health issues, it also damages family relationships. Many women find it hard to forgive the mother or aunt or grandmother who stood by while they were being cut. And then, after all this, being somehow 'blamed' for not enjoying sex. In the FGM documentary *The Cutting Tradition* one woman summed up the problem when she says, 'If we were not cut, we would welcome our husbands!'

Like a plague, FGM has spread across continents, injuring and sometimes killing women, girls, even babies, and it will take further generations of education to shift these beliefs and uproot this ruinous procedure. But there are signs of a gradual shift. In June 2018, the Somali Attorney General announced the first prosecution for FGM, after a ten-year-old girl bled to death following a traditional cutting. (Let's not forget, the nuanced phrase 'traditional cutting' means holding down a screaming, terrified child while an untrained midwife or local healer slices their labia and clitoris with a piece of glass or a razor.) And in a country where FGM isn't banned, and since 98 per cent of girls there are cut, the fact that the Attorney General is taking an FGM death seriously is a huge step forward.

And the name of the little girl was Deeqa Dahir Nuur.

Amana

'He was as fed up with me as I was with my life,
and the only reason he saved my life, as he told
me, was because he did not want the pain of
arranging a funeral for me.'

I had my first orgasm seven months ago. Right now, the pleasure I felt is overwhelmed by the guilt. I am married, and it wasn't with my husband. I am so ashamed and confused but, most of all, I am just lost. He is married as well, and she is someone I know. We used to be friends, but now I cannot look at her because of the guilt and because I am so jealous of her. He tells me that it's not the same with her and that I have always been the one he wanted to be with, but I rejected him, I chose family and having them back in my life over this pleasure I have experienced and being with a kind, loving man.

My life has been one of pain, so the idea that today I would be talking about a love triangle and sexual pleasure is not one I could have ever thought of.

At the age of one I was subjected to FGM and literally stitched up. My only purpose was, like some kind of human gift, to be opened on my husband's wedding night. I was something to be passed around like a pipe; I was not involved in any of it, I did not even eat or drink during the whole thing. My mother had just passed away and my father deemed me to be an issue, so he wanted to get rid of me, he wanted to send me as far away as possible. From a small village in West Africa I was sent to New York. I had visited London with my mother to get treatment for her cancer, so I knew of New York but, even as a fourteen-year-old, I knew I was not there to see the sights but to become a wife/gift to some disgusting man. I was there to serve his needs, like my father's own young wife. She was twenty and my hate for her was why I was there. When my father married her she made my mum's life hell; she told my father that my mother had hit her and, in turn, my father beat my mother. I blame that beating for her cancer. He beat her so bad she never recovered. Watching her die was so painful; her asking me not to be angry and me lying to her that I would not be angry nearly killed me. How could I not be angry? How could I not want to kill those who hurt her and left me, at twelve, all alone and with no one to protect me? I came back to Gambia raging, and that was when he decided to sell me off, like the cash cow I was.

My first day in New York was spent in a downtown clinic run by a man who unstitched the girls sent across the world to the men in the West. I remember looking up at the ceiling, with tears running down my face. I was not crying because I was in pain or because I was scared, but because I knew, had my mother been alive, this would not be happening. I would be back home, with her and in school.

The so-called marriage lasted months. After being raped and being in so much pain I could not take it any more. Just after my fifteenth birthday, it all got too much and I attempted suicide. I would have been successful, had my husband not come home to find me. He took me to the hospital and left me there. He was as fed up with me as I was with my life, and the only reason he saved my life, as he told me, was because he did not want the pain of arranging a funeral for me. Yup, he was a charming human and he left me all alone in America to find my way. I was grateful for that, as sending me back home would have been worse. I then met some great people who helped me, and 'he' was one of them.

I enrolled at night school, and that is where I met him. He introduced me to his family and they adopted me; his sister and the woman who is now his wife became my surrogate sisters. I rebuilt my life, applied to college and really thought I was free. He and I got close and we fell in love. He was and still is so kind, but when he went to his family they refused to give their blessing. I had been married, I was trouble and troubled. It was so painful to be rejected by people I thought knew me better, but I understood.

He wanted to go against his family and get married, but I knew the pain of being estranged from your family. Without telling him, I left NYC and moved across the country, cutting contact. This was before Facebook and I did not have a mobile either, so there was no way for him to get hold of me. But that is what I wanted.

It was lonely, but I kept busy, got myself a job and made some kind of life for myself. All was going well till I got news that my younger sister, who was now a teenager, was getting married. I knew she would not have the strength to say no, and I needed to go back to Gambia. Walking into the house my mother once filled with love, now cold, was hard. I found my sister still in her uniform, a week before her wedding. She and my brother are my mother's only children and they are all I care about.

I wanted to just run and hug her, but it had been seven years since I had seen her and she was so big, yet still my baby. I had to keep it together as I had to stand up to my father and tell him how wrong it would be to put her through the pain and horror I had faced. As much of a bastard as he was and still is, he is human, and I reminded myself of that as I sat waiting for him to come home. He greeted me with a look of shock. I don't think he was expecting to see me ever again and I am sure he started the rumours that I was dead back in Gambia.

After refusing to hear me out and telling me the marriage had been agreed, he left the room only to come back in and blackmail me. He said if I got married to the man myself and took him to America, he would not marry my sister off and would let her finish school. I agreed – of course I did. I could not bear the idea of my sister suffering. She also had FGM as a baby, our mother was gone, so I had to step in and protect her.

I have now been married to that man for eight years and we have three children. I have never loved him, but I love my sister and, for her and now the kids, I have stayed. I ran into 'him' a year ago. I was back in NYC to do some work. I had never forgotten about him and when I saw him he had not changed one bit. We hugged as if we were teens again – honestly, there was no intention to get together. We just connected, and I even lied and told him I was happily married. He said the same, but I think he was being honest. I grew up with his wife, and she is beautiful in so many ways and happy. Maybe that is what having a fulfilling sex life does for you.

We talked every day for months before anything happened, and when it did I could not have wished for it to happen any differently. He was so gentle, so loving. I think I fell in love with him even deeper. The next morning, waking up next to him, I forgot where I was but, within a second, his smell came to me and I remember my stomach flipping. Will you think I am odd if I told you I have never kissed my husband? Our lips have met, but we have never kissed like people in the West would think of it. But I kiss 'him', I kiss the hell out of him, and sometimes that is all we do. It was all we did before anything else. He tells me I am beautiful and, coming from an FGM-affected community and growing up here, he understands the 'mess', as I like to call it, down there, and how I feel, emotionally and physically. I believed him when he told me I was beautiful, I believe everything he said, but I still am thinking of now having a clitoroplasty, as I am told having a clitoris will help me. I might not need love and to be held, but I can just have sex and even orgasm. That is all I want right now, actually. I cannot go on living without a clitoris and for the man I love . . . it is just not fair. I now know what I am missing, I know how it feels, I know the longing for it. In terms of him, I cannot see him again, I just cannot, I must not, it is going to end so badly. I can never leave this man I'm married to. Staying married to him is the only insurance my sister has. If I stay married, my father will leave her be and she can have the life I wish for her and I know my mother wanted for us both.

I once read that every cell in our bodies is destroyed

and replaced every seven years. I believed this and worked on that to get over my first marriage, the hate I kind of have for this one I am married to, and I am hoping the guilt will be gone in seven years as well.

The cut that heals

Clitoroplasty is the surgical reconstruction of the clitoris, restoring both the outward appearance and what doctors call the 'sexual function' of the clitoris, which is really the function of pleasure. It's a cut that heals after all the pain and misery caused by FGM. As a procedure, it's not that well known – in fact, when I did a spell check, the dictionary didn't recognize the word 'clitoroplasty', offering up 'chlorophyll' instead.

My throat thickens when I think of Amana. I don't want to talk in terms of people who 'deserve' love, because everybody does, but she has suffered so much and, maybe if she does have a clitoroplasty, she could have an orgasm, but I wish her love as well.

Iris

'He walked towards me and I think
I fell in love then.'

I was thirteen when we got married. I was young, even if you looked at the world outside of my village fifty years ago. I am sure there were girls far away who had a few more years to her life, before the responsibilities of marriage and a home to keep.

In my village, I was old, at thirteen, to be getting married. My mother and other girls were all around eleven when they married and at thirteen they had their first baby. It was customary to arrange the marriage of daughters within the first year of their birth and for them to get married when they started their period. But, for me, that period never came, and my family decided not to tell anyone and when my thirteenth year came at the time of the harvest, it was agreed I would be married to the man I had been promised to since birth. My mother was more worried than my father that people would find out that I was going to get married without starting my period and she made me promise never to speak of it. The story was that, as it had not rained and the harvest in the last two years had been so poor, we waited for rain, so our married life would be blessed. When she or I now say 'blessed', she meant 'blessed with children', and many children at that, which of course I hoped for, too, and for years to come would pray and pray for.

I had never seen or met my husband before our marriage, but when I saw him I was surprised. He was young. I had always seen the other girls marry very old, or older, men. It was only those who had money and whose family sent them to school who married someone closer to their age. My husband was fifteen; he was tall, and he was handsome. I remember the fear just washing away when I looked up at him. He walked towards me and I think I fell in love then. I felt okay about it all. We were strangers and, to him at that moment, I was nothing more than the promised wife for as many cows or seeds as his father had offered mine. But there was an ease, as if I had met him before, as if I had known him and his eyes before.

As he sat down next to me so many questions ran around my head, but it was forbidden to talk, even if we were to become husband and wife. The shame of speaking would mean people would label you a whore and my mother would of course die from the shame – not literally, but I was not taking any chances.

The ceremony was so long I think I fell asleep at one point, and he poked me to wake me, and that was our first touch. I looked at him for a second and, as he smiled, I fell in love. That smile is what has kept me going over the years. It is what I see now and what I go to sleep on every night. As odd as the exchange of a daughter for livestock is, our families cared and wanted us to be happy. And we were happy, happy for three whole years. He loved me, and I loved him. On our wedding night we talked for hours, we learned about each other. I had known who his father was and how many siblings he had, but I had no idea what his nickname was, his best friend's name or what his hopes for the future were.

We held hands and nothing else for the first few weeks of our marriage. I am not sure if either of us knew what else to do. But one day after he came back from fishing, as it was the rainy season, as he stripped in the dim light, I saw him look at me differently. That was the first time, I think, he lusted for me and, along with his smile, that look is something that still sends me wild. There is longing inside of me, which I feel deep down when I remember that look. That night we became husband and wife in the eyes of God. It was painful at first, it was sharp, and he kept falling out, or maybe 'coming out' is the better phrase. I did not say much, and I tried to control my face. I did not want to show the pain, but soon it got easier and I could feel myself relaxing, which, as I did, made it easier. It was nice, and I enjoyed it. We both enjoyed it. So much so there was not a night that we would not run off to our room in his parents' house and be together as soon as he came in. My mother-in-law would complain that I was not there to lock her son away and she would tell him that he should be ashamed to be spending so much time with his wife, when he should be with his father and the other men. But he took no notice and we built our world behind the green door which stood on the far left of the house. Neither of us could read, but we would look at newspapers he found and dream of going to the city, getting jobs there and starting our own life. I was so happy, I was so in love.

Looking back, I could not imagine how the man sitting beside me would slowly become the most important thing to me and the sole reason behind my life. There were days when my in-laws pushed him, asking him to leave for the city, like all the other men, and find work alone. But he would not and could not leave without me. We were addicted to each other – his smell would keep me going till he came back – but one evil night those hours turned into a lifetime. He had gone to play cards after fishing. He was not given to drink and I don't know if he had as much as they say, but he was drunk. On the way home, it seems he wanted to take a short cut, and here my mother-in-law blames me for his death, in that he was rushing home to see me. I stayed up till the break of light, creeping into the kitchen. I thought maybe he had slept outside, but he was not there. We waited for hours for news and, that evening, it came. He, the love of my life, was gone. In that moment I passed away myself. My heart and everything else broke.

The funeral was worse than the wedding, in that the aloneness I felt when I was given away soon left me, but in him leaving me for ever I had nothing. My in-laws blamed me, and I was too broken to care. As his wife and still just a girl, because we did not have children, my pain was dismissed. I could get married and have a life, his father would say. But I knew how that would never be and how he would always be my one and only.

One day, out of frustration and overwhelming pain that I was not able to share with anyone, I took what belongings I had in this world. Addy and I – yes, that was his name – we had been saving money, and it was not enough for us both, which is why he was working so hard. It was enough for me to leave and to take a boat to the UK. I was travelling alone physically but I could feel him with me and I think he kept me safe.

It's been sixty years that we have been with each other in spirit, and it has just been us for all that time. I have never been or wanted to be with another man. You look at me as if I am crazy, but the love, sex and pleasure I have learned is beyond the physical. Addy is here with me and, for a long time, our relationship was more about anger and asking why he left me alone, but I have learned he has not. I still see his face, and it might be my hands I use to give me those feelings his hands once did, but it feels the same. He is not a ghost, he is the light in my life, he is the man, the soul, I was blessed to spend my life with.

We have always been just by ourselves. He is on one side and me on the other, but at night and even during the day at times we are together. We will soon be together for good, and maybe that coming together will be even better than when we were physically together, and I long for it but, right now, we are enjoying this winter sun, talking with each other. It is faith in each other and those great moments we shared that keep us strong. So, don't feel sorry for me becoming a widow at fifteen; think of me as blessed for having found the love of my life that can last even beyond the grave and still send me wild. That is what I want you to walk away knowing. The sexual connection we have is beyond this world. You kids would understand more, were it not for porn.

Spirit love

Aeschylus said, 'There is no pain so great as the memory of joy in present grief.' Iris was married for three years and has been widowed for over sixty, yet she maintains a relationship with Addy, her late husband, through her spirit. And it seems that hallucinating dead loved ones isn't uncommon and may help the bereaved person. In his book *Hallucinations* neurologist Oliver Sacks cites several people who claim to have seen and heard their dead loved one speaking clearly, while others have a strong sense of their presence. It's different with Iris, because she had nothing to remind her of him. Most bereaved people will have a favoured object or item of clothing, and some degree of support from other people, but Iris had zero support and nothing of Addy's but her memories and her love. And yet, while still a child, she left everything she knew behind and came alone to England, with only Addy's memory to comfort and protect her. And sixty years later, he is still very much by her side.

Helen

'The orgasm I had that night made me scream.
And even thinking about it now makes my
knees go weak.'

I can't remember my first orgasm. I suspect I had a few before Adam Rollins [not his real name] – now, he was the best. I was twenty-two and had been with my soon-to-be-husband for only three months at the time, therefore, it was not cheating. I follow the rule that all is fair game before 'I love you'. I think we all have relationship rules, and that's mine. I got it from *Sex and the City* so, of course, it's a golden rule.

I met 'Jon', as I like to call him (which he hates), during our first term at Oxford and we had lots of friends in common. We'll be getting married in a few months, after six years of dating, something I really couldn't have predicted. He was nice enough when we met, and I found him funny, but he could also be so boring. I mean, he was forever working, and after two beers he'd just leave the party. After the first year I saw little of him, maybe in passing at events, but just before graduation there was a big house party where people we both knew lived. I didn't recognize him at first, he'd grown his hair and looked less square, but I wasn't very attracted to him and when he asked me out I was honestly taken aback. I accepted because ... well, I mean, I was only in town for a few more weeks and, if he was moving to London, he might be the one other person I would know in the Big Smoke, as my parents called it. (They loved 'Jon', by the way.)

We went out a few times before we ended up in bed, and it was okay. And when I say 'okay', I had what I always thought were orgasms with him. Some kissing, some poking and then crashing about till morning. That was the drunken sex of uni life and the 'do you have protection?' line always broke up the kissing and wandering hands. Thankfully, I'm just before that age where boys all expected a blow-job as something to start the party.

When I moved back home, 'Jon' came too. He drove me up and I went to see him in London once before I met Michael, who'd just come back from travelling. Our first encounter was after we were both on the late shift and stayed back for a drink. I was temping after graduating and trying to find what I really wanted to do. Being back in the Lakes was lovely and life was simple again. But now I could legally drink as well.

I'm not sure if it was the fact I was back at home and felt like a teen again, or that Michael (who I always call by his full name) was the kind of guy I lusted after but never dated, because my dad would have had a fit. Or maybe it was Michael's stories of travelling that spoke to me. Anyway, as we walked home, we stepped into an alley and kissed like teens. I was wearing some super-skinny jeans but, somehow, he found a way to keep them up and yet get his hands down there. It was bloody exciting. Trust me, that moment kept me in wank material for days. I think I would have let him do more there, but someone walking a dog came past.

The first time we had sex was after our co-worker's leaving drinks. I knew it was going to be good, and it was. We went back to the caravan he was saying at. I'm sure if anyone was walking past they would have seen (and heard) what was going on. The orgasm I had that night made me scream. And even thinking about it now makes my knees go weak. In the morning we had tea and went to a restaurant. Over the next few weeks we had sex all over the place. My mum saw him leaving one morning and I got the disapproving 'tsk' and the 'What *are* you doing?' talk. I was just having fun. He was the first and, sadly, also the last circumcised man I slept with. Maybe he could go on so long because he was circumcised, but

I'll never know unless I have a wild few weeks before the wedding, which I won't. I love my fiancé.

I really hope that getting married doesn't make us boring, but I'm sure it will. I moved to London after a few months of being at home. I took up a graduate job in the City and settled down with Jon. Our sex life has evolved, so the nervy student sex is gone, been replaced with care and love. We don't worry about STDs but about getting pregnant, so I went on the Pill. There's no scrabbling in the dark for a condom or worrying about a drunk roommate walking in by mistake. We're happy. Emotional sex and love orgasms are what I have now. There's something to be said about having someone you love and respect in bed with you, someone who might be a bit boring but is lovely and who you love.

I won't lie, though. Michael will forever stay in the wank bank. Who knows? He could 'cum' in useful one evening.

Urgent sex

There's something about upright urgent sex with someone fumbling to get his hands down your jeans that's ten times more exciting than polite bed sex. And then she has furtive sex, with the possibility of being heard – no wonder she screamed. But then she worries about how being married will make them both 'boring'. So, was the sex more exciting because of Michael's skill or because it was all so new?

Sex is in the brain – literally. According to anthropology professor Dr Helen Fisher, when you have sex with someone new or amazing or both (lucky you), your brain fizzes with norepinephrine, dopamine *and* serotonin. Dopamine is associated with reward and creates a sense of novelty, hence making you obsessed with your lover. Norepinephrine puts your body into an alert state, giving you a racing heart, and serotonin is the happy hormone. People with a low level of serotonin are more prone to depression.

But it can't last, or we'd all be rushing round, not eating, hearts racing and shagging in corners. All this early excitement quells after about eighteen months, to be replaced by intimacy – if you're lucky. The stuff that anchors you in a relationship but the opposite of what makes sex immediately exciting – danger, passion and newness.

We hardly ever see long-term sex on telly. Long-term couples chat in bed, or the scene is about the fact that one of them doesn't want it. Most of the sex we see is new, and hetero. For some reason, it nearly always involves falling into rooms or the woman being pushed up against a wall. She's never wearing her hideous period pants with mismatching bra and nobody ever farts or trips over their underwear.

Habon

> 'He is – well, was – so lovely that I thought
> saying anything might make it worse and
> knock his confidence.'

I have been divorced for seven months now and being back in my childhood bedroom is odd. Not only because

I am not a child, but because I have one myself now. I am thankful that I have somewhere to come back to and I don't regret getting married so fast. I guess it was meant to be and I was meant to have my son.

We got married and moved overseas within a month, so the excitement of all the new things kept us going. We lived in Mecca for the first few months and I made friends easily. I did need him to go out and get things like the shopping done, but I was happy with that, as it was what I signed up for. When he was not around and I could not leave the house I could invite the sisters I had met over to keep me company. Life was good, we were good.

The first week of our marriage we spent in London, getting used to living together, as I had never kissed a boy, let alone lived with one. I was on my period the first few days, so we did not have sex and I ended up losing my virginity in the Holy City. We had both prayed the final prayer of the day and got into bed. He said a blessing and we asked God to make our union a healthy, happy and joyful one. When all you know about the man you are in bed with thousands of miles away from home is his name and family tribe, having sex for the first time can be a tad overwhelming. Maybe also because he was nervous, it was fast, and he did not look at me much. I did not look at him either, really. I might have been twenty-seven, but it was like two teens in bed. We went right to sleep after that first time. I had hoped he would cuddle me, but there was none of that, he just turned away. This might have been okay if he was some old man who grew up in a place where that was not the done thing. But we were both born in the UK and he is a London boy. He should, even if he, like me, had not dated anyone before, have known that women like to be held. I was worn out, not from the sex, as that was over in ten minutes, but from all the travelling, and being in a new place meant my sleep pattern had not settled yet.

Next morning, we woke up, washed in the way set down in Islamic law after sex, prayed and got ready for the day. It is odd, how uncomfortable he was with just talking about general stuff and being a couple. I knew he was shy, but we were husband and wife now and I wanted to talk, joke and be a real couple. He was very formal with me and even getting a kiss was hard. But I prayed on it and realized we had only been married for a few weeks, I had started bleeding on the poor boy on our first night in bed, so maybe it was understandable.

I come from a family where we are very open. My dad knows when there is a crime scene in my pants and stays out of my way. So if, by mistake, I leave my criminal underwear in the bathroom, he knows to just bin them or put them in the wash. I would always say, 'Put them in the wash,' even if they will never be the same, but my dad, being a man, will bin the ones you know are from a night when your pad has moved, or your period was such a surprise that you had to change the damn clean sheets you put on two days ago.

I wish I could say the formality between my husband and I eased as time went on, but it didn't, so I learned to adapt, just as I learned how to get pleasure from the very formal sex we had. We were married for five months when I had my first orgasm. I am not sure whether I gave myself the orgasm and he was just there, or if he did. I had learned his moves and knew what was coming next. For weeks I could feel myself climaxing and, just before I got there, he would finish and fall asleep. Yup, my thirty-one-year-old husband would finish within fifteen to twenty minutes and fall asleep. I did not show my frustration or say anything, I just prayed for guidance and strength.

He is – well, was – so lovely that I thought saying anything might make it worse and knock his confidence. It was not that he was bad in bed, it was just that he was the only one having fun. At least, I *hope* he was having fun, as I have never spoken to him about it, but just learned to work around it, like I said. I found making noise meant that he would slow down, maybe wondering if he was hurting me, or maybe he would realize there was someone else in the bed taking part as well as him. But it worked, sort of. I did not go too far and sound like – well, those sounds they make in films. I am not sure I've ever watched porn, but I have come across the whole 'yeah, baby, oh yeah' groans, along with the 'OMG, just there, ooh, yeah, yeah.' There is another one I can tell you, even though I have heard it I have not used it in bed and I don't intend to.

Him slowing down and even looking at me meant we got a connection and I had some time. That was nice. There still wasn't the passion I longed for but, when we connected, I finally had the full pleasure of a married sexual relationship. I am not sure if the passion was something I created in my head or something natural. That, because I was now married, my body released some kind of freakish or hormonal need for intimacy. But I still had this longing for more.

Our son came along a year after we got married. I was happy to have someone else at home with me while my husband was away. Someone who, when I loved and cared for them, I could see it *meant* something to him. It was the connection.

We had little sex after the baby, not because I had lost my sex drive, but I just could not stand the emptiness of it all. It takes a lot out of you to be next to someone night after night and give so much but get next to nothing back. When we did have sex, I hated myself afterwards. He would always fall asleep, in his own world, while I lay there next to him, feeling used and cheapened. The sex was not out of duty, it was honestly because I wanted it and, after a few weeks, even after childbirth, I had needs, but the aftermath soon became too much to even allow myself to feel horny.

I started to feel dirty and hated myself for it. I found it hard to look at myself, let alone him, after sex. Self-hate is like a cancer. It starts in one place – for me, the bedroom, and being in bed with someone who had no interest in my happiness – then it began to consume the rest of me. Outside the bedroom, we used to get along, watching TV, reading and learning Arabic together, but soon the idea of even being anywhere near him made me sick. The cancer of hate was everywhere. I had crossed the world for this man, I had trusted my life and my soul to him. But he was just a selfish ass. I would find myself looking at him at times when we were out or in the living room, wondering what I had done to deserve this, or asking as I prayed for God to show me the lesson I was meant to learn.

Nothing came and, eventually, I just left. I left because I could not handle the anger raging within me and I knew that not only did our son deserve better, but so did I. I have been back home for a few months and I don't miss him. I have not told my family the real reason we broke up and I am working on being happy again. Of course, I miss sex, but not with him. There is a fire within now whereas, before, it was just a light. Now, sadly, it is burning bright. I say 'sadly' because there is no one to feed it or put it out.

I am still married. Our divorce is not final, so I cannot date, because that is not allowed, and I cannot marry while I am still married. You will tell me to please myself because, basically, that is what I did when I was married. I worked on getting myself off then, but now I just cannot bring myself to do that. My son also shares the bed with me as well, so if I have maybe thought about seeing what it would be like to get a hand down there, seeing my sleeping son has stopped me.

We will see what happens. I am aware that I will not lock myself away for ever and never have the God-given right to sex, love and pleasure, but right now I am not sure where to start.

Selfish in bed

As Germaine Greer said of bad sex, 'because their penis gives them so much pleasure, it is difficult for them to imagine that it is not doing anything for the recipient of their attentions'. I didn't talk to Habon's ex-husband, and he was probably unhappy in the marriage too but, clearly, she wanted sex and wasn't turning him down. He just seemed locked into his own little world. And they couldn't talk about it, so, you might say, their inability to communicate was down to religious repression. But there is an Islamic Marriage Handbook with whole sections on sexual technique, on foreplay and just how important it is to pleasure your wife. So he couldn't claim ignorance. I'd like to see another world religion with such detailed and useful information about actual sexual pleasure. A Catholic friend said the only nuts and bolts she could find on 'the wedding night' (and this was after pages and pages of 'how not to sin') was some guff on how 'one might compare the physiological side of marriage to a flower that takes time for all of its radiant petals to unfold'. Thanks. Really helpful.

Faith aside, what makes a man bad in bed? Like those blokes who think that saying, 'I've had sex with 350 women,' makes them sex gods. No, it doesn't, it makes them so crap in bed that nobody ever wants seconds. Not incompetent or clumsy – that can be gently dealt with. But bad in bed always means selfish. Always. I mean, come on, guys. All you have to do is pay close attention to her and stop rubbing so hard. You are not cleaning the cooker. A light touch in life and sex is a good thing.

Goldilocks

'I couldn't believe that I had walked into this poor guy's house with a vibrator and a chicken kebab, told him I had been faking for the last few months and passed out.'

I am so sore. He is the biggest I have ever had so far, but still no orgasm. I am now the Goldilocks of dick in search of that golden moment – not too big, not too small, but just right. I'm not sure what the issue is. I can and have come with a vibrator. I have never put the vibrator inside, but it does do the job.

Since moving to London I've not been afraid of dating a lot of men and I've slept with who I've wanted and when. Over the last year, I've slept with a lot of people. I used to think I couldn't come with a man because I lived in a small city and the guys were so unadventurous. So yes, I thought I could come to London and find someone who would help me come *in* London.

When I first had sex I was very young and I had no idea what I was doing. I was shaking as we did it. It wasn't exactly painful, but my head was full of so many questions and fear. I was seventeen and at college, the boy was someone I went to high school with. I really liked him, but he was always with someone in school and I was not allowed to date. My parents are not Victorian or religious people, they just thought it was not a good thing for my sister and I to date while we were in school. It was fine with me, I wasn't that interested in boys anyway. I was a teen, so I had crushes. I kissed boys, but never went on non-group hang-outs with boys.

When I learned that John was at the same college and hadn't stayed on at sixth form either, it was so exciting. He was one of the few people I knew in this massive complex that was a major college in Bristol. He was a smoker, and I wasn't, but I would hang out with him, talking about the school day, bands and stuff, and it just developed from there. On a fag break one day, he asked if I wanted to come to a house party at his place. His brother was back from uni and they were having a party. I said 'yes', trying not to sound too excited, but I was. It would be the first house party that I had ever been to and his brother was so cool. I'd met him a few times. He was in the same class as my sister and she had dated his best friend, so I'd seen him a few times outside of school looking like a boy-band member.

Because I'm a loser, I got to the party at seven because he said, 'Get there around seven.' Apparently, the phrase 'Get there at seven' means 'Get there at ten or eleven.' I was the only one there apart from John, his brother and some of his new uni mates who had stayed over. Cringe! I hung out with their mum in the kitchen for a while and she left around nineish, so I went to join the guys, who were drinking beer and playing music. I sat next to one of the uni mates, and it was easy to talk to him. John was lovely – well, he still is, from what I see on Facebook, and that night was beautiful. It wasn't his first time and that meant I hoped he knew what he was doing. But what John did and, to be fair, what *most* boys did was to basically put their stick in the hole. He said it was because he had a few beers beforehand and that was why it was so fast. I suppose it was okay, I was just yucked out by the mess. There was a lot of mess and I still have an issue with sperm. Imagine if women made that amount of mess! I had been on the Pill for a few months for acne and we should have used a condom for more safety, but we didn't. STDs didn't cross my mind – just not getting pregnant and we had that covered – but had I known how sticky and disgusting sperm could be, and the quantities of it, I'd have insisted on a condom. You can see that the idea of pleasure or orgasm was not something I was thinking about. I don't know why but I just assumed no one had an orgasm their first time. No idea where I heard that or why I took it as fact, but I did. It was only after meeting my first proper boyfriend when I was nineteen that I started to get concerned about the lack of orgasms or climaxing after sex. I had been seeing Alex for four months when I told him that I had never had an orgasm. I was drunk, and I had come back in from a night out with some of my uni mates. (I had decided to stay in Bristol for uni, so I would catch up with old mates when they came home.) My best mate had invited me to an Ann Summers shop, which, oddly enough, was next to the biggest department store in the city. The drunker we got, the more sexual the conversation became and, between the fifth vodka or maybe the seventh, I told Hannah that I'd never had an orgasm with a man. I told her I really liked Alex, but after months of nothing but a cuddle, with little mess, as he knew I hated sperm, so he used a condom, I was bored. That word 'bored' seemed to really shock Hannah, so she marched me to Ann Summers. As we pulled the door open we were greeted by a woman with pink hair. Hannah told her why we were there and then she showed me all the vibrators before pointing out the best one. 'This is fucking amazing, it will get you off and you can keep Alex for the rest.' I bought the pink vibrator.

It was funny at the time but, in the taxi home, I got myself really worked up. I was nineteen. I was not ready to give up and settle for a vibrator when I could have a warm body *and* a bloody orgasm. I walked into the bedroom, where Alex was fast asleep, and started kissing him and trying to undress myself. It was Tuesday and he wasn't a student, so he wasn't impressed. He switched on the light and was really pissed off. The look on his face was WTF and he pushed me away and stormed off to the toilet.

By the time he came back I was in tears and his face had softened. He asked what was wrong and I just let it all out and told him that I needed orgasms in my life. The poor soul had no idea what was going on but, through drunken weeping, I pulled out my new toy and said dramatically, 'I want *you*, not *this*, to make me come.' Then I passed out.

I remember waking up the next day in a pair of his boxers and alone in bed. He had gone to work, and I was hit every five minutes with flashbacks and an overwhelming desire to die. I couldn't believe that I had walked into this poor guy's house with a vibrator and a chicken kebab, told him I had been faking for the last few months and passed out.

The idea of seeing him again was too much so I took myself, my vibrator, the toothbrush and the tampons I had left there for those moments and ran for the hills. We didn't have many people in common, so avoiding him was easier than you think, but it still was hard – fucking hard. The idea of seeing his face and remembering what happened was enough to keep me away from half of the city.

My pink mate the vibrator and I have got very close and I have been able to give myself my first orgasm, but I haven't been able to put it inside. I'm too scared for that and it's not fair for me to expect a man to match the vibration of a battery-powered Made in China toy.

I came (ha!) to London with so much hope. There was a little tingle down there from weeks of playing with myself and my toy. I had bought matching underwear and I was ready to meet some real men, maybe even some who had read *Fifty Shades* and not freaked out. I had given up on the idea of love and relationships and it was all about sex. I was open to everything and I'd slept with everyone, but still nothing. I haven't even come close. I haven't given up but, being almost thirty now, I think I can accept that maybe it might not happen. If a trip to a swingers' club, girls-only events and basically standing on my head during sex hasn't done it, I don't think anything will work. I really like this BIG guy, he is smart and funny, so maybe I am finally happy to settle for that.

I do enjoy the sex and I get wet, I just don't finish, and I can't say I'm missing what I've never had. If I had an amazing sex life and lost it, that might be more of an issue, but as soon as we're done talking here, I'm off for a curry and a cuddle on the sofa. That will sound sad to some but now I'm just not chasing that holy moment. 'That OMG Moment', as you called it when you explained this chapter. I can live with it, I can be me and I have accepted that this is the best I will know.

Faking It

In a 2017 survey of 2,000 people across Europe and the US, 68 per cent of straight women said that they faked orgasm with their partner, and 59 per cent of gay women. As for men, the figure was 25 per cent of straight men and 48 per cent of gay men.

If the true size and scope of the clitoris was only fully discovered in 1998 by Australian urologist Helen O'Connell, and we know that about 70 per cent of women orgasm by clitoral stimulation, I think of all those millions of women who thought they were 'frigid' because they didn't have a vaginal orgasm. Goldilocks thinks it's not fair to expect a man to match a vibrator. Fair enough.

Getting a quick orgasm from a vibrator is no match for the deep sense of intimacy you get from making love with a partner who takes time to pleasure you – it's incomparable.

I have a sneaking suspicion that what often happens is, like Goldilocks, you really like someone, the sex is a bit 'meh' and you fake it, hoping it will get better. It doesn't, so when the hormonal horny cocktail wears off and you're still faking, your partner assumes everything is okay, and it gets harder and harder (sorry) to sit them down and say, 'Well, actually . . .' And then resentment creeps in, which really is a passion killer.

Fato

'I do know that I could live without sex, but why should I? Sex allows me to take ownership of my body and explore and express myself as a woman and sexual being.'

I've been taught that sex before marriage is forbidden, a massive sin which will send me straight to the fiery pits of hell, or at least somewhere as bad. I say, 'somewhere as bad', as hell doesn't always have to be hot. I'm told it can be cold or, like Earth, only full of more horror and pain. This is something I've grown up with and, sadly, something I believe in. The fear of it has led me to marry for pleasure and not love or security, which is something big in my community. I enjoy sex and I'm also a very good student who has learned a lot about my faith or, well . . . the culture of the faith I've been brought up with.

I pray, I fast, I give to charity and I have sex. These things are all part of my life. Each one gives me comfort. Practising and learning Islam helps me create my own morals and ethics within the narrow framework of my culture. I'm not as Islamic as perhaps I should be, but I've learned to be okay with this.

I first had sex at the age of eighteen, on my wedding night with a man chosen for me by my father and his family. I did mind that he was much older than me, but that just seems to be the way it always is, and he was very rich. He had never married and was good-looking for his age. He looked after himself and, because I was so young, he knew I had never been with anyone before.

Our first night was great and he seemed over the moon. He enjoyed the fact that, having never been touched, everything he did to me was not just new but also excited me. I had no fear of my wedding night, unlike many women here that I know. They seem to think that men are monsters and, yes, they can be, but they can also open doors to amazing experiences. In my culture, like many others, women are meant to bleed on their wedding night, as this is meant to prove you are a virgin. I'm not sure if the blood droplets on our bed-sheets after three days of sex were from my hymen or the fact that we had sex for days non-stop. It was painful after a while, but I enjoyed most of it. His commitment to keeping fit was paying off, as after the first night I wanted more and more. I had no idea what an orgasm was, but when I first came, which now I know I did, his face was a picture. He was so proud of himself. I was just flat out, it was as if I had blacked out for a few moments. I was hooked, and I wanted more as soon as I regained my senses. I remember the confused but pleased look in his eyes. I had read that pleasure was one of the key gifts a marriage gave you, and Lord, it did just that.

Beyond the sex, my husband and I had little in common. He was old and boring. He was closer, and still is, to my father's age, but if we could have great sex, I could carry on with my studies and not think of children for a few years. I was happy. He, too, was happy with this. After all, he had a young woman who wanted him every night and did not object to trying new things in bed. New things within reason, that is; there are things forbidden, even for a husband and wife. He understood this and did not attempt such things, which is something, if I am honest, I was worried about. I did not want guilt or the fear of hell consuming me, like the time I had a dream about a boy in my class. That boy was so beautiful and all I did was think of him and me lying next to each other. I was unable to control my mind that night and he came into my dreams and, may God forgive me, maybe I have seen his face in the dark while in bed with my husband. But the Devil is forever around, and I pray for forgiveness, which I hope I get. You can see I am consumed by guilt and fear of being punished for being as sexual as I am.

I would not say our marriage was bliss, but it worked well, and we got on for two years. Just before our third year of marriage, my husband was diagnosed with cancer.

It was in the prostate and it had to be removed, to save his life. The treatment was hard but we came to London and he got the best of the best and, thankfully, he was okay, but there were complications. I was not with him when the doctor gave him the news, but because of the surgery he was unable to get an erection. He did not tell me any of this and maybe I would have been readier for it, if he had.

At first, I tried hard. I really did, and for months, after he got his energy back, we tried to have sex. He was never big on oral sex, but he gave me more to keep me happy. We looked online for things we could do and we tried them all. It was not the same, though. I needed a full sex life, like we had before. I was honest with him and my family.

I was told by my mum I would be a devil woman, as divorcing on grounds of sex would have people talking. But I didn't care – he married me to have people talk about him having a younger woman. He was not ashamed to tell them how he kept me happy in bed and that I liked it, so now I wished for that to continue. My faith gave me the right to seek divorce on those grounds and I wanted to exercise that God-given right.

I do know that I could live without sex, but why should I? Sex allows me to take ownership of my body and explore and express myself as a woman and sexual being. I'm comfortable with my curiosity and I know my rights. Within the laws that governed my life, many of them stopped me from doing so much more, so now I am using ones to empower myself. The role of a woman, be she the wife, daughter, sister or mother in Islam, is well defined. The duties that are placed on us are ones we deliver, but few ever seek to find out the rights we have. Rights which outnumber many of those in any Western country.

Since the divorce, I have moved to the UAE and I have been remarried for a few months. My second husband is also older than me, but not as much as the last one. My family are happy with the marriage – well, they have no choice: I had to leave Doha because it was so small and the only men who came for my hand were men with other wives. They wanted me as a trophy, the man who married the woman so-and-so could no longer please. That is not me. My body is to be pleasured as much as it is to give pleasure, and that is how it should be.

Not talking about erectile dysfunction

Fato is an amazing woman. She wants a full sex life and isn't prepared to compromise. But I did wonder what would happen if her second husband developed erectile dysfunction, not because of prostate cancer, but just by being older. And how would they deal with it? We're always told how important communication is, but if you google 'erectile dysfunction' and 'my husband', what comes up are pages and pages of 'he won't talk about it'; 'he won't admit there's a problem'; and 'it's ruining our marriage'. I spoke to a friend whose boyfriend is older than her about this delicate issue. Even broaching the subject is tricky. I mean, we chat freely about periods, cystitis, the sudden, sinister appearance of pubic hairs above the belly button, but how to ask about her boy-friend's penis performance? We were in a noisy bar, and I blurted out, 'Does he ever have trouble getting it up?' rather loudly, which coincided with an embarrassing lull in the conversation at the bar. But she told me that yes, he does (he's sixty-five) but because he's brilliant with his fingers and tongue it doesn't matter to her, though it does to him. 'He says it's very common in a man his age, but he won't go to the doctor, and ED can be a sign of heart disease. But also, he'll get a hard-on and then, halfway through sex, he'll lose it and get very disheart-ened. And then he'll spend time trying to get it back, getting more and more anxious and worked up. I really sympathize, but there's also a part of me thinking – just go to the fucking doctor!'

A man can walk into a doctor's surgery and stroll out with a prescription for Viagra, while it takes nearly ten years of suffering, on average, for a woman to be diag-nosed with endometriosis, as Tasia found earlier. So why don't more men go to the doctor? It makes me think about male fragility. If the centre or the 'root' of their male prow-ess doesn't work the way it should, it seems to wreck them.

Faith

'I cannot count how many times I have cried after sex because of the pain I feel physically, so any notion of an orgasm is something I don't even think about. My life is what is on my mind.'

I have been married for a little under a year and, before that, I had dated, but nothing sexual ever. I was overweight as a child and a teen, so I did not get looked at, really, and the boys who did look at me were as socially awkward as I was so all we did was drink hot chocolate and hold hands, at best.

I met my husband two years ago, just after I finished university, and instantly fell in love with him. He came up to a networking event and I think he could see how nervous I was. We got talking and soon found out that we had a few people in common. Coming from a BME background in somewhere like Sweden, that is not an odd thing. I really fell for him – he was religious, kind and handsome (to sound shallow). When he offered to give me a lift home that evening I jumped at it. We worked not far from each other, so we started having lunch. He was very accomplished and had his dream job and his life all planned out.

The fact that he was very religious, but not in an overpowering way, was something I found really attractive. He knew so much about our faith but was not judgemental, so he knew that I smoked and did not pray but accepted it. He would tell me things about how the faith was accepting of people and it was all about doing things at our own pace.

I am currently in a post-graduate nursing programme and will be graduating next year. I took this course because of his support and faith in me. I was confused as to what to do next when I met him, but he was older and had been there and done it all. He told me how he had wanted to be a dentist when he started university but changed and now is a chemist.

We dated for a few months before he told me that he wanted to spend the rest of his life with me. I was over the moon and jumped at it again, like when he offered me a lift. My family was pleased as well. He was so respectful, and I was so happy. He really cared for me and wanted the best for me. That is what I thought, anyway. We had kissed, and that was it, he said he respected me too much and I was to be the mother of his children, so he wanted God to bless our home and therefore we should wait. This made me feel so special – I really was walking on air until the day we got married.

I was born in Sweden so, trust me, I know about sex and relationships. I fancied him so much that it was hard to stop myself from jumping on him, but I wanted to keep it special. He was excited as well, I could feel it and see it. We never spent the night together when we dated, and he would always have me home at a respectable time. We dated as Islamically as we could.

The night after our wedding we stayed at the hotel. We did not have sex until the next morning. I remember how happy I was and how what I dreamed about that day is so far from what I have now. That morning we got up, prayed, asked for our marriage to be blessed with happiness and health. We made love after, and he joked and said, 'Do you think we just made a baby?' I remember the grin on my face was only secondary to the glow of happiness that filled me there and then. I am not sure if I had an orgasm, but I was so happy, I think the whole wedding day and night was one long orgasm.

It all went downhill from there. What went wrong? I am sorry to cry, but it is so painful in so many ways. My beautiful, smart and (I thought) caring husband is a sexual sadist. Right after we got married he changed. We did not have sex the first few nights in our new house, as we had family who came and stayed for the wedding. But as soon as they left he started to act strangely in the bedroom. It started with him being very rough and biting me.

I was very confused at first and tried to go along with it, but that was a bad idea. He got more aggressive physically and the sex started to hurt. He choked me a couple of times and, at one point, I thought I was dying. I started crying, and only then did he stop.

The next morning, he apologized and promised me it would not happen again. He told me he had been waiting to make love to me for so long he got carried away. I accepted this because I thought this was the guy who would not hurt a fly, the man who was so kind and who everyone loved.

That night it started off okay. We kissed, and he told me how beautiful I looked, but just as we got down to it his hands went around my neck, and when I asked him to stop he slapped me, and I thought I was going to pass out. He said some of the most disgusting things I have ever heard, and I just started crying, but he did not stop. It was as if something had taken him over.

*

He always states that he cannot control himself during sex and, because I am so sore for a few days afterwards, he is different when we are in bed and not having sex. He keeps saying he won't hurt me again, but I am too scared to take his word for it.

I have developed anxiety when it comes to sex because I fear for my safety. I have screamed or tried to scream for him to get off me, and he can see he is hurting me, but he carries on. No, I have not seen *Fifty Shades of Grey* and, ironically, he would say it was sinful to watch it, like what he says about porn. But I *know* he watches porn, because the stuff he wants to do is not normal. Those things do not come into a God-fearing man's mind.

I get nervous and anxious every time he kisses me. I cannot count how many times I have cried after sex because of the pain I feel physically, so any notion of an orgasm is something I don't even think about. My life is what is on my mind.

Choking in porn

Rule 34 is that, if it can be imagined, then it exists in porn. And among the violent subgenres is a newer trend for choking women. And it's edged its way into the mainstream by being rebranded as 'breath play'. Which sounds much sexier than squeezing the trachea so hard it causes loss of consciousness (which can happen in five minutes) or shoving a penis into a woman's mouth while she chokes.

Even in BDSM, which is all about consent, safe words

and trust, breath play, or auto-asphyxiation, is considered very dangerous, as so much can go wrong. And in that scene, the idea is that restriction of oxygen increases orgasm. But if you see a porno featuring a man having sex while choking the woman, that's not about increasing orgasm, it's about his power and control.

In domestic abuse, a woman might be kicked or punched, but it's strangulation that's the biggest single indicator that your abuser will kill you. Police will arrive to hear the man admitting he 'choked' his partner, which doesn't sound as bad as 'I tried to strangle her.' And most of us assume that, if someone dies from strangulation, it happens at the time. That's not the case, as even though there might not be massive bruising, the woman can die later from respiratory complications like pneumonia, blood clots on the brain, or what's called Acute Respiratory Distress Syndrome, which can lead to fluid in the lungs. I doubt that Faith would describe what her husband does as 'breath play.'

Ellie

'Now I spend my time wondering if he'll want
me to piss on him or snapchat my ginger pubes.'

I've been living in Dubai for three years now. I'm from Liverpool originally, and then I lived in London for a year or so, when I saw this hosting job advertised. I had a pretty good idea what 'hosting' would consist of, as they were paying up to $2,000 per week. When I landed in Dubai I was tanned and had waxed all my ginger bits, but now I'm pale as fuck and ginger carpets are my cash cow. I've not had an orgasm for months. The men I meet are either too sexually repressed or so twisted that I'm too busy trying to stay unhurt to think about orgasms. I miss them, I miss having sex for fun, fancying someone and just wondering what it will be like. Now I spend my time wondering if he'll want me to piss on him or snapchat my ginger pubes. Some of them are good-looking, well educated and not as messed up as others, but I'm still just a piece of meat to them, something to show off and not a real person.

I lost my virginity very young. I was fourteen, and it was fun and games with one of the boys in the upper-sixth form from the local boys' school. Like many of the girls at my school, I had sex and back-street boys on the brain. My first time was fast and uncomfortable, but I liked him, so I didn't hold it against him. A few weeks later at the summer ball, we got to give it another go. This time it was in a bed and we had a conversation beforehand. He thought I was fifteen, and I was going to be in three weeks, so I didn't correct him. His kisses were soft and, when he moved his hands down my body, they weren't shaking. I was overcome with excitement, not nervousness. The orgasm wasn't exactly mind-blowing, but like this warm feeling all over my lower body which led to me just wanting to smile. I must have looked like a total dick, but I just wanted to grin! He had that effect on me and, over the years, we would meet at clubs and, knowing we were each other's firsts, it would be special, and my stomach would flip when he looked at me.

Only one other man made my pants tingle while he was across the room and that was because he had the controller to my vibrating underwear. Harry was not my first love, but he had something I miss so much – trust – and I also liked him. I don't trust many of the men that I meet and, even when I'm drunk and in the mood, I can't get that feeling in Dubai. My brain just won't stop overthinking and assessing whoever I'm talking to. Thing is, when there's money being exchanged then, for sure, there is no connection, and I will not be cumming. It's sad, and I'm not sure if it's been worth it, despite the money. So, when I go back to London in a few months, I am done. I will be able to buy a house, which is the real value of all this time here, but I'm not sure if I can undo or get my mind back to where it was before I got here.

Before, when I lived in London, I could go for a night out, dance, go home with a hot man and fuck till the sun came up. It wasn't lovemaking, just teenage shagging and one-night stands. But it was fun. After this time in Dubai, though, the idea is just depressing. Despite the money, I'm in the shit. Literally, sometimes, with piss added in. Sorry to be so disgusting, but I'm at the stage where the idea of sex disgusts me as much as it depresses me. It's all so toxic.

The disgust started not that long ago, actually – I guess it was just me hitting the wall. This city is full of people who are here just for the money and are leaving soon. This is something you know when you land, especially if you're from the West. It's not like it's NYC or LA. Nobody really comes here for *anything* but the money and, maybe because of that mindset, it's not long before you start accepting other things without thinking about it. At first, all I did was party and dick, but then the drugs came and the out-there requests. First it was just this fascination with my hair and skin, then it was getting me to dress up. I was okay with that. But once you dress up, the door to another world opens and I've stepped inside it. And once you have, it's hard to close again.

But I'm lucky because at least I can leave. Some people can't. They tell themselves that the money, the nights out, the lifestyle, the drugs, will ease the pain. From the outside, it does. You get girls having expensive hair weaves, designer clothes – all that – but behind closed doors they weep. I weep and I'm lucky because I'm leaving. But it does something to your soul.

Sex shouldn't be dirty, but here in the big, shiny five-star hotels it is just that. It's empty of humanity, or contact. Sex here is mindless and disposable. If we were all kids on an island for summer, it might be okay. But these are people with power, influence – actual grown-ups – and it is every weekend.

I hope I make it to the end of this contract.

Escort work/hostessing in Dubai

There's a series called *The Girlfriend Experience* which explores the chilly world of high-end escort work. A young law student wants to earn extra money and joins an agency. Lots of shots of beautifully dressed young women sliding out of mirror-polished cars and stalking into anonymous glass buildings. What struck me was that the loneliness in Ellie's soul is reflected in this world of silent, luxurious hotel rooms. There's never anything homey – no photos or books – just huge, anonymous spaces.

The thing about escort work in Dubai is that, once you strip away the glitter, the yachts and the money, you still have a man who's paying to get his rocks off. Only, powerful men who can buy anything seem to get jaded, so women like Ellie end up catering for all kinds of weird kinks. Powerful men also come out with the 'busy busy' schtick, that they don't have time for relationships or intimacy, blah blah, but most of them are married. It's power and control in exchange for the loss of intimacy.

Ellie said that she wanted to make it to the end of her contract, but she never said whether it was because she was worried about being injured, or losing her ability to enjoy sex, or just the emptiness. I really hope she makes it and gets out with her soul intact.

Bea

'I can say that I have a great sex life and I do have orgasms almost every time I have sex, but this has come at a cost and being empowered

has meant that a lot of men feel threatened or
emasculated by my self-knowledge.'

I had my first intense sexual dream at around eleven. I
shared a room with my younger sister at the time and
I was so worried she might have heard. I knew what it
was, as I was always playing with myself; it was warm
and comfortable between my legs. My poor mother was,
of course, horrified by this. She tells me to this day how
she was called into my nursery school because I was
always putting my hands between my legs during story
time. I wasn't wanking, for fuck's sake, so I've no idea
why they felt the need to call my mum.

I'm a teacher now and the boys are forever in the
playground with at least one hand down their pants.
Well, maybe not their school pants, as they're a tad tight,
but any given day there's a young boy in a tracksuit, hands
down his pants, blissfully playing with his balls. I'm
okay with this – don't get me wrong – I'm sure it feels
fab. I just don't get why me doing the same thing was
such an issue. I'm sure boys in the 90s were as busy with
their hands as they are today.

Back then, I knew that my intense dream was a sexual
one and the feeling I had was an orgasm because, a few
weeks before, we'd gone to the beach and, when we
came back, my mum told me to make sure I washed the
sand out. I've no idea why, given where my hands usually were, and I hadn't put the shower head up there
before, but to get the sand out I certainly got busy with
the shower head that afternoon. It tickled at first and I

stopped right away, but then when I tried it again, it felt amazing. All warm and wavy; it just took over my body. I wanted that feeling again and, when I did it again, the next morning, I intentionally pushed it right up there and again it was delicious. I still give thanks to the power shower and do it occasionally. It's a forceful but pleasurable feeling.

I have no idea how that feeling ended up in my dreams and felt so real, but it did. I don't remember what I was thinking, but it was so real. If I was a boy, let's say I would have wet the bed.

I'd consider the dream my first orgasm, but along with that I've also had other orgasms while awake and fully taking part. So, I suppose I've had several first orgasms. Knowing how good the shower felt and how delicious it was to have a hand on top of my vagina, I got to thinking what it would feel like if I put my hand in there (or, more realistically, a finger). I took it slow, as I was a bit scared. It was the weekend, my mum had taken my sister to a play club, my brother and dad were out, too, so it was just me in the house. I was meant to be studying for exams, but I needed a break and just got into bed. Closing my eyes and just exploring; it was so warm, wet and lovely. When I came it was like my body was melting out into ache, like the cat when she brings up a hair ball. I was light-headed and just fell asleep. It was only when my mum came home and started calling me that I got up.

The sensation of cumming is so intense for me – I still find myself blacking out for a second. That sounds a little fucked up, saying it to someone who has had FGM. I am sorry, but that is how it just feels.

It goes from the physical to the mental. I think of that little blackout as some kind of reset. So when I am stressed, upset or need to get off to sleep, an orgasm can fix all that. This can be from sex or a wank.

The next orgasm on my 'first' list was with my friend Laila. You see, all that studying post my first wank paid off and I got into a great all-girl school. Don't worry, she wasn't some girl I'd met at school and started talking sex with. We'd been childhood friends and she was very aware of my sexual ways. We'd been talking about pubic hair and how mine were very much darker than those on my arms and legs and I asked if this was the case for her as well. That is how it started. She wasn't sure, so we agreed that we would have a look after school. Mum was always happy to see Laila anyway. It was just meant to be an informal session about pubic hair, but then she asked about where I touched myself to get these electric shocks I'd been talking about.

There in my room, with my little sister's stuffed toys looking beadily on, we pulled our pants down and explored. I showed her where I liked to touch myself. She wanted to touch herself as well, so we looked for the same spot on her body. We were both almost thirteen around the time. There was no kissing and, even though I had my little 'O', which by now had become a friend, things with Laila weren't sexual. We could talk about anything. She wanted to know what worked for me. It was innocent, and it would be others who walked into that room who would have made it sexual. *If* anyone had walked in.

Unlike me, she didn't masturbate, but I loved her for being that friend who never judged me and the one who didn't have any bush till she was in her late teens.

For someone who was so sexual, you might think I'd have sex early, but I waited till I was at uni. Knowing what I liked and whereabouts I liked it made it easier to enjoy what turned out to be a very drunken first experience. I think I did most of the work – he just worked the equipment.

I soon upgraded from him to the guy who ran the union bar. He was one of those guys in their twenties who thought he was a fresher. He did, however, give me the first orgasm where I didn't have to direct everything, like a plane landing on the runway. It was good, and it was also my first multiple orgasm. This was well before porn so, thankfully, there was no flipping unnecessarily, just the right amount, moving to positions I had no idea of but he knew would get me there and, boy, they did.

I can say that I have a great sex life and I do have orgasms almost every time I have sex, but this has come at a cost and being empowered has meant that a lot of men feel threatened or emasculated by my self-knowledge. When I was younger it was a real issue, as guys my age who I liked thought I was 'too forward'. It was their insecurity, of course, so I found myself sleeping with older men. They were usually more okay with someone who knew what she liked, although some thought they could teach me a lesson or two. Hmmmm. They did that occasionally, for sure, but I also felt kind of used, as if they saw me as a way to relive their youth and at the same time teach me a few things which would, of course, blow my mind.

God is watching and He's disgusted

My friend Siobhan tells me that her thirteen-year-old daughter learns about consent in sex-and-relationships education but still nothing is said about female masturbation. When I was learning sex ed, she says, the emphasis was very much on self-protection. Be careful about contraception, be careful when you go out, watch your behaviour. My mum used the phrase, 'Don't go and get yourself raped.' But if girls don't feel free to explore their bodies and learn what feels good, and if you add that to this bizarre idea that men are supposed to somehow know what to do, it's a recipe for really rubbish sex. Of course, it's important that girls and boys are learning about consent, especially with the prevalence of porn, but there's still very little emphasis on pleasure, particularly on girls pleasuring themselves. But, aside from masturbation being natural and healthy, it teaches girls what they like sexually.

Religion and masturbation are a touchy subject (boom boom). There is nothing in the Bible that explicitly forbids any masturbation – the story of Onan is about him 'spilling his seed' after coitus interruptus, thus, any child born would not be his. Apparently, God was watching (hmmm) and slew him. Whereas the Jewish Talmud forbids male masturbation, as it leads to 'impure thoughts' and spilling semen, there's nothing about women. The Quran takes a slightly different view. While it's generally permissible for spouses to masturbate each other, the attitudes to solo love seem to vary depending on the Islamic scholar you speak to. Some say it is *haram* (forbidden), while others merely refer to it as *makruh* (disliked). The religious right in America take a far more po-faced attitude. Not only have they released videos and books entitled *Every Young Man's Battle* and *Every Young Woman's Battle*, tees are available from a group called the Passion for Christ Movement, or P4CM. Yes, you too can walk around wearing an 'Ex-Masturbator' T-shirt and be the envy of all your friends. And the Jehovah's Witnesses released a sign-language video about the evils of masturbation in which a young man barks: 'Jehovah is watching, and he's disgusted!' Wow – God watching *again*? Does he really have nothing better to do?

Of course, it's always about control. If you can control somebody's sexuality, you can control them. You won't be surprised to hear that use of online porn spikes very highly in the Bible Belt.

Female masturbation has a long and lubricated history. Greeks used breadsticks lubricated with olive oil and, centuries later, vibrators were invented to 'cure hysterical women'. In fact, Dr George Taylor invented a steam-powered vibrator, to aid something that would get a doctor struck off immediately today.

While men routinely arrive in A&E with Hoover hose stuck in eye-watering places, women more sensibly have taken advantage of the bouncy spin cycle on the washing machine. So, you can get your clothes dry and get yourself off at the same time. Way to multitask, ladies.

The Manipulator was invented by Dr George Taylor in 1869. Are you turned on yet?

Anni

'I have had an orgasm, but it was more just breathing for the first time.'

For years I prayed that God would answer me. I did not and would not have sex until I got married. I love that you will not and have not laughed at me. To say in 2016 that I was a virgin until a few weeks ago is odd. I am white and middle class. I live in London and sex is everywhere. I have worked and prayed so hard to keep true to my faith. Being a Christian is not cool and dating has been bloody painful.

I met my husband about a year ago. Telling people that shocks them and they think we had some sort of movie-style romance, which maybe we have, but I think it was God's doing. My husband was in town for a few weeks when we met. He works in oil, so he lives in the Middle East. He saw me in a coffee shop and came over to ask if I minded him sitting next to me. I did not, and we just started talking. We exchanged numbers and spent the next two weeks together. I admit that finding out he was not a man of faith worried me and I waited for him to try and kiss me and then seek sex, but he did not. Many men will try to kiss you after the second date, and when you say no, they never call, or they question your faith and commitment. It is very trying. I love God and I know He had a plan for me to meet my husband, but He has tested me. I did kiss my husband before we got married. It was the day we got engaged – but you want to know about the sex. Well, the fact that he was travelling for the year we were together before we married meant it was easier physically, but not mentally.

I am not sure if he really did not sleep with someone else when we first met. He said he didn't. I do believe, in the end, he came around, knowing how important it was to me, and he wanted to be with me.

The night before our wedding I prayed that all would go well and that I would be enough for him. I was worried because I have had issues with my body. I developed an eating disorder when I was fourteen. It was finding God that saved me from the disease, but it has also meant that now my organs and bones are messed up. I have the weak bones of a seventy-year-old. Knowing he is used to women who are healthy and experienced really worried me, and it still does.

But despite my fears, he was so loving, and I need not have worried, but I did anyway and still do. We have sex every day since we got married, and it is beautiful. It is everything I prayed for. His love for me is in every part of the whole process. We have not done anything out there yet. I think he is holding back, and I will find a way to tell him. Because our year together before we married had not been sexual, we did not even have a sexual text exchange.

Before my husband, the last man and only man I have loved broke me. I could not give him sex, so I gave him what else I could to keep him. I said things I did not believe in, I moved away from God. When that was not enough, he left me and the darkness came. I did not look to my family or God for help. Instead I went back to Anni, which is what I call my eating disorder. She is always around and, when I met my husband, I was in her grip, but he has been superhuman to hold out and he has freed me from her and the darkness. I hope I can make him happy and get over the issues I have. In God's eyes, we are man and wife and nothing is forbidden. Nothing should be between us. I do love that he does just lie next to me and I feel so open to him, but he has seen the world and I still worry I might be too boring for him. He is a hot man and women who are better looking and smarter than me are out there. I have had an orgasm, but it was more just breathing for the first time. Not having sex or even trying anything sexual has been like holding my breath for thirty-odd years. Now I am married, the feeling I get is one of letting go and not a high. After sex it is messy – I don't like that, but I also don't feel guilty. Sometimes, when I would look at him or my ex and think of them naked – just naked, nothing else – I would feel so sick. I would pray for guidance. Now I just pray that my husband is happy. In the coming weeks I hope we will find out more about ourselves, I pray that God will guide us. My husband does not care much for God, but I am praying a lot about that. It is only with God that we can make this work, and I want it to work. I have waited so long for him and all this love. I love him so much and I need him in my life.

Sex after anorexia

Many women who have struggled with anorexia also report problems with intimacy. Sex with another person is, as Anni (also the name she spoke to me under) has said, messy, and involves letting go, relaxing and throwing yourself into pleasure, whereas the world of the anorexic is the opposite. Rooted in control, an anorexic girl often strives to be perfect and ordered. Many have rules about food, such as the peas can't touch the carrots, or that absent-mindedly licking a cake spoon means two hours on the treadmill. This behaviour drives their families mad, but the sufferer believes these rules keep extreme anxiety at bay. Having an eating disorder feels as though an emotionally abusive partner has taken up residence in your head and is constantly telling you how ugly and fat and useless you are.

Beat, the UK eating-disorder charity, has a section where sufferers have their recovery stories and I was struck by Anni's comment about learning to distinguish your real self from your anorexic self, because surely the first step towards sex with another person is acceptance of your body, yourself. Anni takes comfort from God as well as her husband, but I felt most hopeful about her future from her comment about how the feeling she gets 'is one of letting go and not a high'. I hope that she can continue to let go.

3. Pregnancy

'I graduated from law school nine
months pregnant.'
— Elizabeth Warren, US senator

'If I had kids, my kids would hate me . . . They
would have ended up on the equivalent of *The
Oprah Show* talking about me.'
— Oprah Winfrey

'Hello, I'm Mila Kunis with a very special
message for all you soon-to-be fathers. Stop
saying, "We're pregnant." You're not pregnant.
Do you have to squeeze a watermelon-sized
person out of your lady hole? No.'
— Mila Kunis

'Yes, I'm positive there's just one baby in there.
Can I throat-punch you now?'
— Anonymous

Pregnancy. Like everything about women, there are so
many assumptions made. For a start, if we don't want to
be pregnant, ever, then there must be something slightly

wrong with us. As more women stop hiding and pretending, instead choosing to speak their shocking truth of just not wanting children – calling themselves 'childfree' – the parameter is starting to shift, but there's still a way to go. If you're a woman and don't want a child, you are still seen as violating unwritten societal norms. 'Selfish' is the favoured insult, or variants thereof. But then, if you're pregnant and decide to end it, you're also being selfish (and heartless). Ditto if you have only one child (selfish and lazy), or more than three (selfish and greedy), or if you don't breastfeed (selfish and vain because you're trying to preserve your perky breasts, *obvs*) or if you breastfeed for longer than a couple of years (selfish and weird).

While some of us fear pregnancy, others long for it and others may have chosen it as something they never want to do, but we do all want to hear about it. So that was how I originally started this chapter, but, like much of this book, during its gestation it changed. As a pro-choice feminist I'm super-aware that as much as the world wants to sell women this vision of the perfect puke-free, varicose-vein-free, alcohol-and-cheese-free pregnancy, followed by the perfect birth and an empowering natural instant bonding, then straight back in the size-ten jeans post-pregnancy, it's nothing to do with the reality for most women. And motherhood itself is hard. No let-up, no time off, full-on judgemental remarks from anyone and everyone with an opinion – and all for free. And these remarks, usually framed as 'helpful', can come from medical staff, parents, friends, strangers, the man in the dry cleaner's, your other children and inanimate objects. (A friend of mine says that her printer 'hates' her because it knows when she's been up all night with the baby and it refuses to print. The printer, not the baby, she adds. We'll give her that one . . .)

I don't have children but, looking around at my friends and in-laws, the disconnect between the fantasy and the bodily-fluid-squirting reality is a mile wide. Whatever you might think of Kim Kardashian, I admired her for being brave enough to say she didn't enjoy being pregnant. 'I just always feel like I'm not in my own skin,' she said. 'It's hard to explain. I don't feel sexy, either – I feel insecure and most of the time I just feel gross.' She'd struggled to *get* pregnant, so how very dare she not eulogize on the marvels of her beatific state? You'd have thought she was letting all women down. But I thought she did the very opposite, and the more that famous women are honest about these periods of female commonality, the better.

My friends tell me that the only reason to have a baby is that you want one so badly that none of the very sensible reasons for not wanting one matter any more. You'll know, they say. You'll just know.

I don't know yet.

So, this chapter ended up being about pregnancies rather than babies. I wanted it to be more about that moment you are staring at the pregnancy test, your life on a precipice, everything depending on whether the second line appears. The twisting and turning of the pregnancy stick – is it *really* a second line or is it the light? – holding it up to the window, or to a light, then seeing the cool scientific evidence of human chorionic gonadotropin, or hCG, in your pee. And that's it. Yes, there is a second line. Pale, but, yeah ... you can't be a bit pregnant. And then a decision needs be made.

This is a decision I have yet been forced to make.

So, as you can see, pregnancy is not simple. That first experience takes many forms. This chapter will look at women's experiences from the twentieth to the twenty-first century across the world. As much as you can read or be told about what to expect, each of us has and will have our own unique experiences of our first pregnancy. Like all the other chapters, this, which is common to all women, is a uniting and equalizing act that shows, no matter where you are from or who you are, we all have a first.

And as this section is about pregnancies and not babies, this chapter will look at those women and girls who have chosen to have an abortion.

Helen

'My sister hasn't had children yet. I hope she
does, and I really hope I can hold her hand like
she held mine.'

It was 19 December 2003. The day of my abortion. I remember getting to Euston and shaking with fear but pulling myself together. I had to come to London with my sister because my GP was a total dick and wouldn't refer me to a clinic. I was twenty; I'd been stupid and forgotten to use protection, just once. But the way she looked at me you'd think I'd been shooting up right in front of her.

I got pregnant at uni but didn't find out till I came home for Christmas. What a present. But it was more complicated. I'd come off the Pill, as it was affecting my ability to focus at uni and I was getting bad headaches. The campus medic told me it was fine to stop and just to play it safe, that my period might take a few weeks to come. 'Don't worry,' he said. I didn't play it safe enough, obviously. I couldn't believe I'd be so unlucky that the only time I had unprotected sex I would get pregnant. But I was, and I did.

I remember paying for the test with my Boots points as I had no cash and for some reason I thought someone would find my statement. It makes no sense, and I am sure I was hung-over, so nothing made sense that day anyway. Maybe I was in shock. I was meeting my twin sister, who was also down from Leeds for our usual 'It's from us *both*!' Christmas-list-planning session. We played the poor students and joined forces on the Christmas expenses. The truth was we wanted the money to get pissed while we were down from uni.

I did the test in Caffè Nero and then just shoved it in my bag and forgot about it. I was so sure it would be negative. Telling myself firmly that I was going to get the coil and never take such a crazy risk again, I got out of the loo and saw my sister. We had arranged to meet and catch up before hitting the shops. These were the times before flat whites were a thing, so we both had a hot chocolate, giggling about the term and boys and going home. I remember because it was only when my sister made a joke about eating for two that I remembered the test. I pulled it out, ready to tell my sis another funny anecdote. But then I saw these two bright pink lines and my gut flipped. I was pregnant. Of course I was. I dropped the test back into my bag and tears spilled down my face.

Looking back, the signs were already there, but I didn't want to see them. I couldn't. When I got pregnant ten years later for the second time, I had the same telltale signs. The sight of white wine would send me into a dizzy spin, the smell of meat would have me running for the loo, and eggs were all I wanted to eat. It's a bit like being hung-over, which may be why I mistook the signs. You feel sick but you want to eat everything you see at the same time – well, all you see that is not milk-based, when it came to me. I'm sure there's some biological setting that you want what's good for your body even when you don't normally want it.

But to go back to that awful painful moment. I am lucky I was in the West and I had my sister with me, but I also know my mother had always said that, if I got pregnant, she'd march me down to the abortion clinic herself. I knew she would be so disappointed. She and my father had worked so hard to get my sister and I into the best schools, they took us on the best holidays, gave us the best of everything, and here I was, about to risk it all. We were the first in my family not only to go to university but we had both got into the one my mum could only have dreamed of. I don't want to sound like I was forced into the abortion, or I didn't have much of a choice, but it wasn't that simple. I didn't want a baby, I certainly didn't want to be pregnant, but I also didn't want an abortion, nor did I know how it was going to happen. I couldn't just pop into my GP and confide in her either. She was the family GP, and she knew my mum. I knew she wouldn't tell her, but I couldn't be sure. She might accidentally let it slip. I also didn't want our family GP looking at me when she saw me at the supermarket or just crossing the road. I thought of waiting till I got back to uni, but that was weeks away. So my sister came up with the solution while I was crying into my hot chocolate. She explained how I could call up my student support officer and organize an abortion back in London. My sister was very relaxed about it. I never asked if she was talking from experience or just making it sound okay to keep me from falling apart. I was in a real state, so I'm pretty sure that's what she was doing – trying to keep me calm. I hope it wasn't the case that she had an abortion and didn't want to tell me about it. That really would have killed me, as we share everything. –

Even though we're twins, my sister was always the risk-taker. She was far more likely to have been in this situation, they would say, and yet there she was, comforting me and helping me to sort out an abortion. 'They' being the world, the world that stands in judgement. My sister questioned the world, she drank, she partied and she would be the one you would never ask to hold the key or the taxi money on a night out. So of course she would be the one to get knocked up but, instead, it was me. Maybe that's why she was so chilled. Defying expectations.

There wasn't any 'cultural' pressure, there would be no shame or the things I heard friends talk about when we were growing up, but there would be disappointment. My mother would be disappointed. I know I was, and I still am. I should have known better, and I have learned from it, but it was a painful lesson.

I had to have a surgical abortion, which isn't as major as it sounds, but they do put you under. I was too far gone for the medical one. But they still told me about it; it meant taking two pills a day apart. That sounds simple, but it would cause a miscarriage and the woman told me it was painful, so I was lucky I only had the surgical option. It all went well, and my sister and I were back on the train and home the same day. I stayed in bed the next day, but when I woke up covered in blood I knew something had gone wrong. This time, going to London wasn't an option and I was too embarrassed to tell the doctor what had caused the bleeding, so my sister rescued me again. She really took care of me, and I love her for it. She told the doctor what had happened, and it seems that, as rare as it might be, complications after abortion sometimes happen. I'd suffered what's called 'an incomplete abortion' so there was still some tissue left, which caused the bleeding. I desperately wanted to ask if the abortion would affect my having kids in the future, but I couldn't.

Why? Because I didn't want to be judged. I mean, who was I to talk about kids when I had just had an abortion?

I've come to terms with the abortion and don't regret it, as it was totally the wrong time. I know that I made the right decision. Thankfully, it didn't stop me having children and I now have beautiful Bella. I'm so thankful for her and feel I was given a second chance. My sister hasn't had children yet. I hope she does, and I really hope I can hold her hand like she held mine. It will be her first pregnancy, it will be so different to mine, but our love and respect for each other will be the same.

Abortion

Following the 1967 legalization of abortion in the UK, anti-choice groups peddled the idea that abortion would give you breast cancer (no, it doesn't, says the World Health Organization) or that you would end up with something called 'post-abortion syndrome' (which doesn't exist, says the Royal College of Obstetricians and Gynaecologists). Later, these groups changed tactics and adopted a faux-feminist idea that *they* were the ones who really cared, and that by standing outside clinics, making it even more distressing for girls like Helen to go inside, and thrusting leaflets containing dubious 'statistics' or plastic foetuses into their hands was, in fact, 'counselling' them. Currently, only 37 per cent of the 1.64 billion women worldwide of reproductive age live in countries where abortion is unrestricted. And twenty-six countries ban abortion entirely, not for rape, not for incest, and not if the mother's death is likely.

There's one thing I've never understood about

anti-choice activists. If you ask them bluntly what they really want, the inevitable response is that they want to make abortion 'unthinkable'. Because stating, 'We want to ban it,' apart from making them sound a bit less 'caring', won't stop abortion, and they know it. Countries where abortion is banned also tend to be far stingier about women's health services, including access to contraception. This means of course that while rich women can bribe doctors, poor women have no recourse or options. Information gathered by the US Guttmacher Institute for reproductive health in 2018 demonstrates that abortions have dropped significantly over the past twenty-five years, but only in developed countries. And what about developing countries? The same report says that unsafe abortions have *rocketed*, and that 'legal restrictions only increase the likelihood of abortions being done unsafely'. Something pro-choice groups have been saying for ever.

Yasmin

'The pain I felt that night in the kitchen and for
months later, which is still part of me, was
reality hitting.'

My husband is gay. I can say that without crying now. My husband is gay, and I live in a prison-shaped mansion. I wish I could say he told me, that he broke down telling me out of respect and love for me and our family.

No. It was the driver who told me and the whole house, just days after I gave birth. I am not sure where he is now, and I don't care. I did care for a while, and that came in the form of hate and anger for him. We were asleep – well, in bed, anyway, as no one gets sleep after a baby is born. My body was aching, as I'd had an emergency C-section. It hurt to move. Suddenly, there was this loud banging on the front door, because the driver had the code to the main gate so he could come right to the door. That gate cost more than some people's flats and it was meant to keep us safe. I say 'meant to', but it's not much use when those who hurt you are the ones with the code in the first place. That driver had access to the code, my door and my husband. I still remember the deep tearing pain as I struggled out of bed and inched down the stairs. My stitches still hurt. It took me for ever at the time but, knowing what I do now, that time seems like a blissful state of being. I was a mum to a baby boy, my family and in-laws were over the moon, my life was set. I could hear shouting as I walked into the kitchen. My husband was trying to push our driver into the back garden, but he was drunk and pushing back, screaming. I had no idea what he was saying at first but when he saw me in the room, he yelled, 'Has he told you how I gave him all of me and how he loved every minute of it?'

Those words were not the ones that rang in my head for months. The ones that did were from my husband, telling me how happy I made him. I believed him. I never asked where he was all those nights when I was alone in our big bed. I really didn't mind the being alone. I thought he was working; he needed to work, he was running a multimillion-dollar company. But it seems he wasn't working. He was with his lover – our driver.

I fell to the floor as he drunkenly screamed and yelled and my husband tried to shut him up. It took me weeks to get up from that fall. The bed became the floor. I stayed in bed for weeks, not eating, not showering, just crying.

The baby was taken care of. We had a nanny, a nurse and all I could have asked for. But there was nothing for me, nothing at all. My husband tried to talk to me, but I could not listen, I did not want to hear it. Our first year of marriage, our first baby – it was meant to be blissful, we were meant to be happy, but it was not. I was in pain physically and mentally. I was on medication and alone.

I could not talk to my mother or anyone else, I did not have the words. My father would demand I left, my mother would never be able to show her face and my husband would not be able to live with it all. I could not do that to my son. And as much as I hated my husband for what he did, I could not sentence him to death. Because that is what I would be doing, as we live in the United Arab Emirates, and sex with another man, under Article 354 of the Penal Code, is punishable by death. I was okay when we got married knowing that he experimented. All the men I knew did that. When you come from such a strict society as ours, it's the done thing. Dating women around the world, drinking, drugs and parties – it is what the men do. But when you get married, that all stops, or it's supposed to stop. Okay, maybe

I am lying there. As the wife, you hope it all stops. But for 'it' to come to your house like it did, and for it to be something deeper than sex, that is what really hurts.

When I finally talked to him, our son was six months old and my mother was flying in to see him for the first time. She had moved with Dad to America just before our wedding and I was so ill during the pregnancy I could not travel. My mother is an amazing woman. She speaks seven languages and had worked for a fashion house, travelling across the world. There is an image of Middle Eastern women as being submissive and kept. But many of us are out there and we have the same issues as other women. My husband had been coming home every night since that night, he spent time with the baby and I think, some nights, he cried as much as I did. He was, and is, boxed in with expectations, to be everything that his father and the world around him wants him to be.

I asked if it was just a fling or if he was attracted to men, but deep down I already knew. The sex we had was never passionate and when I told him I was pregnant it was as if he had done all he needed to and we became like siblings having to share a bed because the whole family was over and there was no space. I say that, as I shared a bed with my brother when we lived in London and the family would come to visit. I did not mind my husband not wanting to have sex, or even holding me, as I had bad morning sickness, which should be called 'twenty-four-hour sickness'. Sitting here wondering about what it was like to be pregnant, it hits me that it was hard. I was sick and struggling, but it was okay because

I was so happy. I was excited, despite the sickness, the swollen feet, the wind, the constipation; everything was okay because I had this guy everyone would kill for, the amazing house, and people were still talking about our wedding, so it was all worth it.

The pain I felt that night in the kitchen and for months later, which is still part of me, was reality hitting. It was the nine months of pain, the twenty hours of labour, the C-section, the loneliness, the emptiness that was my pregnancy and is now my life.

When I asked my husband how it all started, he tried to make excuses. Eventually, though, he admitted that he had been seeing the driver before we got married and hoped that getting married and having a baby would change things. He thought it was just sex and that he had looked for help, but it was deeper. He was happy when he was with him and anxious when he was with me. He was honest and told me that, as hard as he tried to love me, he just could not. You would think hearing that would break my heart, but my heart had been broken months ago. It had been so broken I was unable to smile when my baby looked at me with brown eyes full of love and hope. I was so grief-stricken that seeing my brother for the first time in months filled me with fear and not excitement. I am now sitting here, and I'm empty and not crying because I don't have the energy left to feel anything at all. Being numb is what keeps me going. It is what is going to help me raise my child and stay married. I am going to stay married, as I am not interested in people talking or asking questions if I move away. I am going to stay married because I want another baby. I want a brother or sister for my son, I want him to have someone he can feel love and comfort with. I will be married in name and on paper. I will just not be married in the way we – well, I – had wished.

I don't care what he does any more. I know he will find someone else. Maybe the driver is still around, maybe he will travel the world and see things I hoped we would see together. Right now, I am this shell, you see. I'm like one of those Russian dolls – with another human inside who will come out. Or maybe there is nothing left to come out.

When being openly gay is a death sentence

Being a gay man is still a criminal offence in seventy-two countries round the world. And under Sharia Law, in Yemen, Iran, Sudan and Saudi Arabia, it carries the death penalty. In Somalia, being gay (whether you are male or female) officially carries a three-year jail sentence but, in reality, it can mean death.

In 2016, a young Somali activist was outed as gay. Thinking that she was going to be married, 'Sahra' was flown to Mogadishu, but while the village elders were in her granny's house a young cousin whispered that they were planning to kill her. Luckily, she had alerted people and, through a relay system of cars and faithful friends, she was smuggled out of the country.

My heart breaks for Yasmin, and her sense of betrayal. But what she is really upset about is the fact her husband had an affair and fell in love. It just so happens the 'other woman' is a man. She was aware that men 'experimented' before they got married but thinks 'all that is supposed to stop when you get married'. But your sexuality is at the core of your being, so how can you be expected to just put a lid on who you are, essentially?

Cultures all over the world have tried to make laws to restrain and control human sexuality, and it never works. From parents sending their children to 'gay conversion therapy' camps, to slut-shaming women, to Islamic extremists throwing gay men off buildings, whatever the penalty, you cannot legislate human love or lust. As Willa Cather says in *The Song of the Lark*, 'The world is little, people are little, human life is little. There is only one big thing – desire.'

Tanya

'The only man I wanted a baby with.'

I am thirty-five and a widow. That word is not something I have heard in my life, let alone it *being* my life. But that is how the world sees me. I am still angry, and for a while I was angry at him. How could he leave me? How can I be where I am now? Right now, though, I am just angry at the world, and especially God, who is the only person – or deity – I speak to, so now, He gets the brunt of my rage.

I was not raised with religion, but the week before

Jem passed away I found myself in a church for the first time since school. I had spent weeks in hospital by Jem's side, weeks trying to be strong, weeks trying not to cry in front of him, holding it together. In that quiet, peaceful church . . . well, it was the first time I started to think about all that would be gone when he left me. That was the first time I thought about children. We had got married young and children were on the cards, but we wanted to get the house, maybe travel and then have the kids. We planned for at least three. Jem was an only child and there are four of us. I would have had a football team with him. He would have been an amazing father.

We started trying a few months before his cancer came back. Jem had leukaemia as a child, but he had been okay since then. Then it crept back. It started with him thinking he had a cold and feeling under the weather, and I thought nothing of it. Why would I? It was his mother who came over and said he should go to the doctor. Jem was an only child because his mum wanted to give him her full attention when he was ill and, when his father left, she never remarried. I am not sure if she even dated anyone after that. For the first time, I was thankful that she was so involved in his life even when he was grown and married.

Jem and I were still very hopeful when we found out. After all, apart from the fucking cancer, he was young and healthy. But the cancer was so ugly and fast, it took hold of him like a forest fire. But we still tried to have sex. We were still trying until the night he was admitted to hospital. I joked about it – the last joke I think I made. 'I had sex with my husband and almost killed him!'

He went to sleep with a headache and later that night he was rushed to hospital and into intensive care. In the morning I left him for a few minutes to get the morning-after pill. We'd been trying but, now, suddenly, he was so ill. I thought he would need me – I could not be pregnant when he was so sick. I am not sure if I would have gotten pregnant anyway. We never had before. I took the emergency pill.

And yet, sitting in that quiet church, all I could think about was that I might have lost my chance of having a baby with the man I loved. The only man I wanted a baby with. I was living on no sleep, so I was not thinking straight, and that is where the anger with God comes from. It seemed so cruel. I remember screaming. I am not sure if it was out loud or just in my head, but I remember rocking and weeping. I asked Him why He did not stop me. Why was He taking everything away from me? Past, present and, now, a future.

Waking up alone is the worst, with no one there to care for. It is selfish, but I wish we had got pregnant, so I could have not just part of him here but also someone to care for and someone to need and love me. I loved cooking and looking after Jem, before he was ill and even when he was. Now I have nothing.

I am not sure if I will have kids. My clock is ticking, but I really don't care. It won't be with Jem and I am not interested in meeting anyone else now. My family thinks

I need to move on with my life, but I have no idea how. It takes every scrap of will I have to just struggle through the days and go to work. The idea of forming a relationship is unthinkable and the notion of a first pregnancy is a myth. For me, anyway. I will never know that, and I know I have a role in that, but honestly, my role is not one I have any control over, even if others think I do.

When you lose the person you love, the idea of what you would have, it is hard to re-create or even imagine.

Posthumous sperm retrieval

In 1997, the Court of Appeal made a historic decision. Seven years previously, Stephen Blood and his wife, Diane, had been trying for a baby when he contracted meningitis. Before he lapsed into a coma, however, Stephen allowed two samples of his sperm to be taken. But after he died, because he hadn't given written consent, his widow was unable to use the samples. There was no legal precedent for this case, and it took Diane seven years before she was finally allowed to undergo fertility treatment in Brussels. Now with two boys, she won a further battle in 2003. Up to that point, there was a blank space on their birth certificates where their father's name should have been. After the Human Fertilization and Embryology Act came into force on 1 December 2003, she was able to have her sons' – Liam and Joel – births re-registered with her late husband, Stephen, as their legal father.

Sue

'Hyperemesis is not just morning sickness, it is
something that has driven many women to end
a really wanted pregnancy, and it has also made
me pro-choice.'

Comparing hyperemesis to morning sickness, or even
calling it that, is like comparing a broken neck to a broken finger. They are both painful, but one is over in a
few minutes and the other means you can't get up at all.
You could say that I was the Kate Middleton before she
became the poster girl for 'morning sickness'. When I
first found out I was pregnant I was over the moon . . .
well, I was, after the shock wore off. I think everyone,
when they find out, whether it's planned or not, can't
believe that it's really happening. You get over that
quickly, I guess, if you planned it like we did and longed
for it. It's then you call your husband at 4 a.m. in NYC
to tell him, and it's then you run down to your best mates
and show them the several sticks you pissed on, before
the shock and disbelief wears off.

Because we wanted this baby/pregnancy so much we
were excited about everything to come. I was excited
about week one, three, seven and sharing all that with my
mum, my sister and my husband. I remember the first
time I was sick, not because I was ill or hung-over but
because I was with *child*. I say that because I was so excited,
and I was the arse who used that term. It was two weeks

after I found out, so I guess I was around six weeks or so. We went out to celebrate at our favourite restaurant and I ordered ravioli. We had a lovely dinner, came home and, just before we got into bed, it happened. This little bubbling sensation in my stomach started. Out of nowhere, oh God . . . I still remember so clearly that desperate need to get everything that was in my system *out* again. I went to the loo thinking I would just spit into the bowl, like I did the last few times. But this time it was head down the Sam (which is what I called my toilet). The yummy ravioli which I was so looking forward to now decorated the inside of Sam. Where, once, he was pristine white, he was now splattered red and yellow. From then on, Sam and I became great friends. I spent more time with him than with anything else. Or anyone. My husband and I soon got over the idea of being disgusted. He had to, as not only was I vomiting more than I was talking, sleeping or anything else, but I also had excessive salivation, which, if you are interested, is called ptyalism or sialorrhea. I had all the medical terms for overdoing being pregnant. You might also be interested to know that the salivation or spitting is due to my diet. Apparently. The midwife trying to make me feel better told me that, because of my African background, women like me who ate spicy food were disposed to have these issues. I didn't have the heart to tell her that, even though I was Somali, I wasn't a spicy-food kind of girl, but I took it on the chin and let her believe that years of ethnic and exotic cooking were worth the state I was in. I wondered what this midwife would have said to Kate? Too many vol-au-vents?

So, between the spitting and the endless vomiting, my husband and I got ready for the baby. Throughout it all, he has been a rock. It might sound like an evil thing to say, looking at my beautiful daughter, the light of my life. But, honestly, four months in, when it was bad, and I could not even get out of bed and had been in hospital for the hundredth day, it seemed, I really did consider having an abortion. When I see my little girl doing something that fills my heart with joy, I remember that moment. Was I really going to abort her? But it was never that I didn't want a baby – I just felt so terrible, all day, every day. Hyperemesis is not morning sickness, it's something that has driven many women to end a really wanted pregnancy, and it has also made me pro-choice. The idea of someone being forced to carry on with a pregnancy in such horror and endless sickness is torture. The labour, after months of feeling like I was going to die, was a walk in the park, but that was offset by the pain of not being able to breastfeed. This was linked to the fact that I was too weak to do so, and I did not want to push it after pushing for several hours. Between the start of labour and my daughter coming into the world, it was around nine hours. I did not find it painful; I did not have gas and air but I had a light at the end of the tunnel. No more sickness or spitting, and Sam would just be the mate I saw once or twice a day and not my closest friend. I was looking forward to what little sleep I would get as a new mum, but sleep in an actual bed, rather than the cold floor next to Sam, my pregnancy toilet mate.

Coming back to our patron saint Kate, when I found

out she was pregnant again after Prince George, I ached for her. Her body, I don't think, had recovered, because the gap between George and Charlotte was only a year and ten months, but even so, I know her head had not recovered from being so sick. Think of the worst hangover, flu, food poisoning you have ever had. It is all those in one go, and it is non-stop. You can sit in a dark room, but the world will keep spinning; you can avoid food, water, even air, but you will still wrench your guts inside out. Yes, it's that painful vomiting when your stomach is empty but something seems to want to come out. My hell was at least private, though. I, thankfully, did not have to step out with the world and the press watching me. The first time I was hospitalized I came in wearing my class of 2005 hoodie. I think it had some sick on it. I had not washed my hair for a week, and let's not mention the bags under my eyes. When I stepped out a few hours later, I looked even worse. The idea of photographers shoving a camera in my face . . . I think I would have puked on them and then died of shock.

Hyperemesis

We're more aware of the misery of hyperemesis thanks to the Duchess of Cambridge. But, as with endometriosis and how long *that* can take to get diagnosed, hyperemesis can also be met with indifference, if you're not royal. According to the charity Pregnancy Sickness Support, up to 1,000 women a year are forced to terminate wanted pregnancies because they are *vomiting up to twenty times a day*. One woman reported dragging herself to the doctor's, where she vomited twice in the car park, and was then ordered not to be sick in the waiting room. You can bet the Duchess of Cambridge wasn't treated like that.

We're talking about not being able to keep water down, so women have died from hyperemesis, or rather the dehydration that results. Before the hospital drip was commonplace, the most famous victim of hyperemesis was Charlotte Brontë, who died four months into her pregnancy. There are anti-emetics now available too, but as anyone who has taken them knows, they stop the actual vomiting but not always the dreadful nausea that precedes it. The vomiting, in a weird way, is a relief.

Hyperemesis, in most cases, clears up by five months, (twenty weeks). But that's five months of vomiting constantly. And for some unlucky women it continues throughout the entire pregnancy. So, for some, labour and birth come as a huge relief in more ways than one.

Violet

'It's almost as though there's an unwritten rule
that if you don't get pregnant, you are fair
game to be told how lucky you are
"he has not left you"!'

God, am I really going to talk about this? I've been freaking out about it. Of course, it's something I've thought about for the last eleven years of my life – it's the elephant with Dumbo ears in the room, at every wedding or social event I attended after my second wedding anniversary, because I would be asked the same questions. I understood, and still understand, as painful as it is, when they ask, even now, why I don't have children.

Coming to the point that I can now talk like this has taken time and pain and thought. At first, I expected to get pregnant, so when people asked, I was flippant, and I would say, 'Oh, give it time.' They would normally also be hopeful and light-hearted and wish me luck or tell me how excited they were about seeing me pregnant soon. When I got married I was only twenty-two so there wasn't much of a rush. But by twenty-five, everyone who had been married as long as I had been was pregnant, or with children; then it started to get harder to brush off the comments. The hope became anger, and I stopped attending weddings, I moved roles at work and the idea of going to my friends' baby showers was unthinkable. I even left Facebook. I was so angry and upset, seeing post after post of babies, their births, birthdays and just being cute little assholes – it hurt so much. My sister, who is only two years younger than me but who got married five years *after* me, when she announced she was having a baby it was the lowest point in my life. I remember when she told me. I was furious how matter-of-fact she was. I know I projected my feelings on to her, but it seemed her announcement was her telling me *this is how it is done.* I was in bed for weeks after I found out, and my mum came over and told me to get a grip and that if I could not be happy for my sister I should fake it. That sounds harsh, and it was, but in pretending to be happy for my sister, I found the strength to be honest with myself. Or maybe I hit the wall that I could not ignore any more. The acceptance of my situation started with getting her to really understand what was going on.

Of course, the assumption is that there was something wrong with me and, to be fair, it was in my case, but the fact that people just assumed that really pissed me off. It was one of the reasons I never went to see a doctor until we had been married for six years, because I had no idea how I would deal with the news. When I found the strength, I remember it like it was yesterday. I was scared that my husband might fear there was something wrong with him and would want no part of it. I wanted to do it together, as a couple, and not just go and get myself checked. He was watching his beloved Liverpool and, as they were winning, I knew I would have him in a better mood.

I'd rehearsed what I was going to say to him. I planned to follow the advice I'd read online, I was going to be all open and non-judgemental. That all went out the window and the words ran out of my mouth. 'Can we talk about having a baby?'

That sounds odd, but before we got married we talked about babies and, after that, having sex was not just a way to express our love but also start a family. I was never on the Pill or anything. A baby was a given at some point. Only it wasn't.

In the six years of marriage we learned to work around my period and not talk about the disappointment, fears or anything related to the fact we were not pregnant yet. We just never talked about it.

When I said those first words it all poured out. No one knows this but, in that moment, I almost said, 'You can leave if it's me.' As much as I loved him (and I do still), I didn't want him to be with me out of duty. He could still have children, if that's what he really wanted. I remember the look he gave me, followed by a kiss on the forehead. Unknown to me, he had been wanting to have this conversation, but not because he wanted us to get pregnant but because he was worried about me. He was worried about the pressure of me being surrounded by people forever questioning me and the state of my ovaries.

The first pregnancy is not, as you say, just about having that baby, it's also the longing for and sometimes accepting it may not happen. It's the odd things that people don't tell you about marriage and relationships. It's almost as though there's an unwritten rule that if you don't get pregnant, you are fair game to be told how lucky you are "he has not left you"! That is the new piss-take – that is such a Welsh term – but the idea that I should be grateful Hassan has 'stayed' with me. Some people assume he should be knighted for not leaving me. That's right – my husband is the first Somali knight and not Sir Mo Farah. Sorry, mate.

I love my husband, and he knows that. I also know that it's not just within our marriage and because of being Somali that the issue of infertility has taken hold and affected relationships. I read the mags and I see the celebs and, being in a small community inside a bigger one, it does sometimes feel like your life is all over the front pages and you are fair game, which is hard.

The results of our fertility tests weren't good, as you might have guessed already, seeing as I don't have any baby pictures up on Facebook. The process, as physically painful as it was, was really healing for my soul. I stopped questioning and hating myself. I found faith in my ability to rise above all the assumptions and expectations. Our marriage does have its ups and downs, but I can honestly say that none of that is to do with the fact we cannot or don't have kids. I'm not going to say it's something I celebrated, but it is something that I accept, and I hope soon others will as well.

Infertility

Violet didn't go into details as to why she couldn't have children. But, with women, the process of getting pregnant is intricate and if one thing goes wrong the whole process is messed up, like fertility dominoes. The woman must release an egg at the right time and it must be waiting in the right place in the Fallopian tube (which makes it sound like the world's worst date). The egg then has up to seventy-two hours to be fertilized. If sperm meets egg, then the now-dividing egg must make its journey down the Fallopian tube to the uterus and embed itself into the lining. So many things can go wrong during this process. The egg might not be released at the right time, or the woman's cervical mucus can be 'hostile' to the sperm, or there might not be adequate hormones to make the uterus nicely spongy for the egg to implant. Sex becomes a grim, carefully timed duty. With men, it's simple: either their sperm is up to par or it isn't. If it isn't, then you can have a treatment where a single sperm is injected straight into an egg. And of course, it's awful if you're a man and the problem is your sperm. It's just that the treatment isn't nearly as invasive as it is for a woman.

The worst is that dreaded phrase, 'unexplained infertility', when there seems to be no particular reason why you can't get pregnant. 'Oh, just relax and it'll happen,' say helpful friends you want to immediately punch.

But what *is* clear is the sheer anguish caused by infertility. As Violet said, she seemed to see fecund women everywhere and it became harder to fake pleasure at other women's pregnancies. And saying 'Well, you can always adopt' doesn't cut it because women feel a literal ache to conceive. Of course, there are hundreds of thousands of children who need a home, but there are far fewer babies, and what Violet wants is to grow and birth and smell and hold her own.

Monica

'I have no idea why people want to share their
horror stories with you, but they do.'

What no one tells you about pregnancy is how crazy you go thinking about death. It took us years to get pregnant. I slept my way through both the high-school and college football team without ever having a scare. I thought I was lucky but, entering my twenties and the world of work, that voice at the back of my mind became louder, but not in a scary way. I just knew and accepted that I might have issues getting knocked up. When I met my husband, a very good Jewish boy, I knew babies would be a thing, if not for him, for sure for his mum and mine. I was not raised in a very religious way. I was more a cultural Jew, so marriage and family was always set as a goal – not the main goal, but up there with getting a house and becoming someone your parents can mention in their annual newsletter. My family still has one, and I blame that for my (almost) breakdown.

When Jason and I met, we had 'the Conversation' as soon as we knew we wanted to be together and before we even got married. I pushed the conversation, like I do everything, deep down. You know, as I sit here look- ing back, maybe I was always so loud and forward with him because I wanted to protect myself from the real- ities of never being able to have a family and being seen as a failure.

Never having had a test, like I said, I still knew our baby would be made in a lab, and I needed him to know that. At first, he thought I was just being over the top, but I needed him to know that getting pregnant wouldn't be easy. I can easily get stressed if I think I'm failing at something, so I like to plan. I saw having a baby as a project. As it was, it only took us two goes at IVF to get pregnant, which meant everyone we knew also trying kept on telling us how lucky we were, and then it all started. In the same breath as 'Yay, congratulations!', there was the 'You should know the chances of a miscarriage' stats. It was the doctor who first started this fucking shit, but I forgave him, because he had to give us realistic expectations, but everyone else could have kept their mouths shut.

I had to give up drinking and smoking, which was a pain and meant I was on edge even before getting pregnant. I wanted the baby so much, but I couldn't relax for a moment; all I felt was fear. Everyone said how 'lucky' I was, but I didn't feel lucky. I felt cursed. I would lie awake at night, tuning into every flutter. I waited every day to lose my baby. I feared every kick was the last one. I cried every day, terrified by this idea that I would be induced, would go through labour and then deliver a stillborn baby, and even then, I would still be called 'lucky', because I was pregnant, so I had felt what it was like.

I don't want to be unfair, but some of the women I met when we started our treatment I can't talk to any more, even though I still love them. The clinic said that talking to someone who knew how you felt was a good thing, but although we all started out in the same situation, some of us were 'luckier' than others. It made talking impossible. Some of us had a baby at the end, and some didn't. Some of us would even have more than one baby, although I have no idea how those women who got pregnant with twins handled it.

I was lucky. I was one of the 29 per cent of women under thirty-five for whom IVF ends with a live birth. I was luckier than the one in a hundred women who have an ectopic pregnancy and a possible ruptured Fallopian tube, which makes getting pregnant again even harder. I was luckier than the one in two hundred women whose babies are stillborn. My head was exploding with these stats all through my pregnancy.

My pregnancy was such a fearful time that, when I gave birth, I was mentally and physically worn out. I was fighting to keep myself from falling apart, and the scream of Abbi was the sweetest sound I have ever heard. If you asked me what my birth was like, I wouldn't be able to tell you. If you asked me what the midwife had said to me during the eleven hours of labour, again I couldn't tell you. All I could think of was that he would not be born alive. That my great-auntie was right, and I would not be able to give birth to a living child because I was not able to get pregnant naturally. I am smart, I have an MBA from one of the top universities in the world, and yet some nasty shit from an old lady who has never left her village overruled everything. The post-man telling me about the horror of his wife going into labour at twenty-two weeks and them not getting admitted because it was a miscarriage rang in my head. I have no idea why people want to share their horror stories with you, but they do. So, all these deaths, near-misses and miscarriages, and it just makes your life hell. My first pregnancy was just death and the fear of death. I'm not sure if I can do it again. I am not sure if my mental health can handle it. So maybe I should just be happy because in the end I was FUCKING LUCKY and have this beautiful bonny boy in my life.

Pregnancy horror stories

Birth is yet another thing that women want to get 'right', whatever that means. One woman remembers being set on a drug-free birth, especially as the woman in their NCT group had assured her that labour pains were 'waves lapping against the shore'. While she and her boyfriend were on a hospital tour, passing the birthing suite, she heard a woman screaming, 'Kill me, just kill me!' and 'Give me drugs, you fuckers!' There was a lull in conversation, the women all looked at each other and the lady taking them on the tour said very briskly, 'Right! On to the wards!' But it's one thing discovering for yourself that giving birth isn't so much lapping waves as a tsunami and another for people to take ghoulish pleasure in telling pregnant women awful stories of childbirth. The writer Libby Purves wrote hilariously of this very thing in her classic parenting book *How Not to be a Perfect Mother*. 'Oh yes, doctor had never seen anything like it in forty years. And it was twin beds from then on . . . the dirty beast.'

The National Childbirth Trust, or NCT, is a great organization and has done an enormous amount in de-medicalizing birth. But if you've had an easy birth, there can be an unfortunate tendency to assume that it's the same for other women, and if they choose pain relief in advance or *clutches pearls* a *C-section* – well, it's just letting the side down, isn't it? Would these privileged women who eulogize the glories of natural childbirth have the nerve to say the same thing to a young woman in Africa struggling through a two-day labour without medical help?

Now that social media is so all-pervading, it has been accused of contributing to tokophobia, a severe dread of childbirth, but maybe it's more about having unrealistic expectations, or a birth plan the length of *War and Peace*, one that you intend to stick to, no matter what. Maybe the real problem with social media is that it doesn't tell the truth. Either it's full of horror stories or it's fetishizing birth with glowing, flat-stomached celebrities (their fleet of staff carefully hidden). To get the truth, you must talk to women on their own. I've never given birth, but if and when I do, I'll probably try and keep my pain-relief options open. It seems that women who are determined to have a certain type of birth, and have idyllic expectations, are the ones who are more likely to be disappointed or feel they've 'failed' when the birth doesn't happen according to plan. As a friend said to me, 'Nobody wants to admit it, but there can be an undercurrent of female sadism with birth. *I* went through it, *I* suffered, so why should *you* get out of it? Well, fuck that. Enduring a twenty-four-hour labour on yogic breathing does *not* make you a better mother.'

Mona

'I was leaking from everywhere, my period had
just come back, or maybe I was still bleeding, my
C-section was like a bloody, smelly zip across
my abdomen, and I didn't have a single maternity
bra that wasn't stained with blood.'

Blood is a lot warmer than pee when it rolls down your legs. I knew it was blood, and not just because I was pushing something as big as a fully grown pug out of my muff. The pain was like a hammer hitting me right in the back and then my body shaking with force. I had my sister with me and it was her face that said it all about the blood. As I pushed like mad, hoping every time it was the last push, this warm flow came. It wasn't as warm as candle wax, more like that first dip in a delicious hot bath on a cold evening. It was oddly soothing. And just like sitting back in that bath, I was overwhelmed by the need to close my eyes. There was no pain, which you might think a funny thing, since I was dying. My sister suddenly jumped back from the side of my bed. I remember her shocked face, and then I blacked out. I'd no idea at the time, but I was haemorrhaging bright red oxygenated blood. I was rushed to have an emergency C-section, and it was touch and go for a few days.

That warm peacefulness was the last time I think I was happy or myself. As painful as the labour was, it all stopped after I blacked out, and I was under for the next few days. I had loved being pregnant, I was excited to meet the little man, and my husband was great. We had just moved into a new place and my sister was going to be the best auntie. I had so many plans.

When I got out of the ICU and was told how lucky I was to be alive, I remember not feeling anything. I just wanted to see my baby. My husband and the rest of the family had been with him since his birth. I was alone in surgery because my sister was too scared to come in and it's not customary for men to come into the delivery room, even if the baby is coming out of the sun roof and not the hatch. We were both in the West, so I've no idea why we believe these backwards things, but we did. Although I'm sure many other women don't want their men in the delivery room.

When I saw my son, Mo, he was the most beautiful thing. Do all the mothers say that? I loved him immediately and wanted to be the best mother I could be. But I was also worried that our connection wasn't growing. While we were in hospital there was support. The nurses looked after Mo, and when my husband came he held the baby and hugged me. I was living in a bubble, one which popped as soon as I came home.

In the hospital, if he didn't latch on to feed, there was someone there to support, encourage and just be there. I had issues breastfeeding and I expected it all to be simple. They say how natural it is, but I found it so painful. And I thought I was failing in the simplest thing. It would take ages for Mo to latch, he would scream, and I would be stressed and crying too. I didn't want to use the bottle. We'd talked about it and my husband, trying to be helpful, would hover over me, telling me to 'do it now' whenever Mo opened his mouth, but it wasn't easy at all. When he did latch on, my nipples became so cracked and sore that blood came out with the milk. He was sucking the life out of me in so many ways, from lack of sleep, lumpy, sore breasts, bloody nipples and the pressure I put on myself.

Being home alone was a depressing environment. I was lonely and felt so useless. I just hated it, and I spent most of my nights cooped up in the dark bedroom. Mo's hungry screams would jerk me out of sleep and I would grit my teeth, knowing how much feeding him would hurt.

The day I broke, I remember standing in the bathroom looking at the mirror while blood was dripping with the milk from my once-amazing tits. I had just put him down. That was the first time I just wanted to die. I wanted peace. I was leaking from everywhere, my period had just come back, or maybe I was still bleeding, my C-section was like a bloody, smelly zip across my abdomen, and I didn't have a single maternity bra that wasn't stained with blood. I'd had this vision of the post-baby life with everything being beautiful, and it had all turned to shit. Standing there, I'm ashamed to admit, I hated my baby, my husband and my life. Most of all, I hated myself. I wanted it all to end, and I came close to doing it with a bottle of painkillers in the kitchen.

Saying this now, it is so scary. If my auntie hadn't come

to the door that day, I'm not sure if I would be here now. My mum had passed away and talking to my mother-in-law was out of the question. She's a lovely woman, but she wouldn't understand. Or maybe she would and I'm being unfair, but I saw how judgemental and traditional she was about some things and she wouldn't understand the idea of struggling with one child when she, as she said, had 'raised five' in harder times. But how does comparing your struggles to someone else's help anyway? I just knew, standing in the kitchen with the painkillers, I was going under.

It was Tuesday, and I had missed my health-visitor appointment, so when the doorbell went I thought it was her. I hid and hoped she would go away, but when the key turned I was shocked. I thought my husband had come back home and I rushed into the bathroom to wash. He used to leave while I was still in bed and he was never back before nine, so he assumed I had got changed back into my PJs when he came back. He had no idea I stayed in them all day, or that showering took more energy than I had. I would have a pirate shower, as we used to call it when we were kids, when I could, using wet wipes and dry shampoo (thank the Lord for dry shampoo). I did the bare minimum so he wouldn't worry. I looked nothing like myself if I'm honest but, then, I had no idea *who* I was and what I *should* look like. I wasn't the professional high-flyer in the city any more, nor the perfect mother I'd planned to be. I wasn't the life and soul of the party. I wasn't even a shadow of any of these.

I don't know when I began my random bouts of paranoia, but I didn't want anyone in the house who might see me as I was. But the fear manifested around the idea that if anyone saw me looking the mess that I was, everything would fall apart . . . yes, like it wasn't falling apart already. But I didn't want to lose my baby, my husband or my home. I'd be in constant fear of something . . . I wasn't sure of what. But I believed it would lead to the unravelling of everything. The fear spiralled out of control and for a time I was convinced that the reason the health visitor came so often was to just catch me out. I was told at pre-natal classes that they called in the first few days when you were home and after that you could come and see them at the clinic every Thursday or make an appointment. But they were calling and making appointments for me, and now I know they could see I needed help.

It was my sister at the door, and she thought we were asleep and had come to surprise me with a visit from my auntie. Looking at me I think I gave my auntie as much of a shock as the day she heard of her sister's passing. She had seen me at my joyful baby shower a few weeks before I'd had Mo, and I'd been glowing and happy, but now I was standing in front of her, a drooping ghost. Those were her words, after I had treatment and got better. I don't think I will ever be better, and that's the thing with mental health and especially when you have a baby. With help and support, you can be well, but words like 'better' and 'fix' are not words I use or find helpful.

My auntie hid her shock well. After we hugged, she told me how well I was doing and how well the baby looked. 'I hope he looks well, he's killing me,' were the words that just rolled out and, in that moment, she said the best words to me. She took my hand and said, 'Success as a new mum should be measured by the fact that you haven't broken any windows or the baby. You're still standing in one piece, so you are the best mother I know.' This might seem like a low threshold for an over-achiever like me, but it was a high bar, a bar it took all of me to achieve.

That evening I took my first bath since I came out of the hospital, and next day we booked me to see someone the health visitor had recommended. I learned that not only was post-natal depression very common, but it was normal and that it was also in my DNA. My mother had issues when my older brother was born. It was something I had had no idea about and something my auntie didn't want to tell me, but knowing about it might have helped. I might have planned things a little differently. I might have been more realistic and not expected it all to be perfect. If we do go for a second child, which I hope we will one day, it will be better because I know who I am now and what could happen.

Mo is four now and starting school. He has no idea how hard those first six months were. He has no idea how much I hated myself, and how his screams would send me into a visceral rage. I hope I never could hurt him, but I'm not sure if that is true. I know I wanted to hurt myself and

I was close to doing that. And I do still think that maybe, as pointless as I am told it is, I wonder if I'd had him naturally, would it all have been different? I don't think so deep down, but the question is there, and it will keep going round and round in my head for ever, I think.

PND

After such a traumatic birth, Mona was exhausted and suffering not only from mastitis (inflamed sore breasts and cracked nipples) but also from anxiety, social isolation and sleep deprivation. And, as well as these miseries, many mothers also feel they lose their identity. Nobody uses their actual name any more, instead they're referred to as 'Mum' and in the third person. 'Mum's a bit anxious,' says the nurse as 'Mum' feels literally sidelined and vaguely foolish. One woman said her biggest bugbear was a health visitor referring to her distress as 'baby blues'. 'I was being jerked awake five times a night by my son crying and for a few seconds would fantasize about throwing him out the window – I was so tired, and she was calling what I was feeling *baby blues*?'

In Mona's case, considering what she'd been through, it would be surprising if she hadn't spiralled into post-natal depression. And like so many mothers, instead of seeking help, she blamed herself. Where have we heard that before? She was lucky that her auntie was able to step in, explain that what she was feeling was entirely normal and get her some help.

Mia

'My daughter is now five and I have seen her
once since she was born.'

I had milk in my breasts when I landed. Well, of course
I did, because I had given birth just a month before I
heard about this job, and a week later I was here in the
Middle East. My daughter is now five and I have seen
her once since she was born. She seems happy, and that
keeps me going. I got pregnant with a boy who was not
ready to get married. When I told him, he left me. My
family is poor, and they could not feed the children they
had, much less be able to keep me and another mouth.

I bonded with my daughter before she was born, as I
did not know how soon after her birth I would be leaving or where I would be going, but I did know I would
have to leave her to make a life for her. I did not know it
was a girl till she was born, but I wanted to share my life
so far with my little angel. It was as if she was my partner during the pregnancy. I did not have any money, but
I had the beauty of the village I grew up in. I would go
for walks with her, patting my stomach and talking to
her about where I grew up, my hopes and dreams for her
and for myself. The closer it got to her birth, I tried to
explain why I would not be around a lot, how I loved her
and, however far away I was, we would for ever be connected. At times she would kick when I was having a
crying fit, scared of missing her so much that I would

never leave. I took the kicking as her telling me she understood. I really hope she does, and I hope it is not as painful for her as it is for me. She has my mother, who is a great woman, and my little sister. My sister was my baby before my baby, and our mother never left. We were lucky – my mother finished high school and ended up getting a job at the local office. It did not pay much but it meant she could stay with her children, watch us grow up and become adults. Her own mother had worked away when she was a child, but only in the City, not worlds away, like me. It is normal for women from my country to be working away in the Middle East. We are the nannies, housekeepers and beauticians. There are a few of us who meet up, and we do talk about our kids a lot. I am the only one who has one child; many others have gone back and, as their husbands are farmers or also work abroad, they set a time and get pregnant. You must be good with your timings.

This is not something I have to worry about. If I do have any more kids, I firstly must find someone, and I have been saving so I will not have to leave again.

The mum of the children I look after is beautiful – she looks like a Christmas tree every day. I am not jealous, because she is also a mother and understands my ache. We are not friends, but she knows I love her child and I long for mine. There are many things, as women, we do not speak of. I don't see her life as easy. I don't see her struggles, whatever they may be, as less than mine. We all ache and we all bleed. She, unlike me, I am sure, does not cry as much, but she worries as much as I do, I know that, and maybe when she travels she longs for her children like I long for mine.

The night I gave birth to my little angel it was raining outside and my waters broke not long after I had gone to sleep. I remember wishing the pain was anything but labour, because it meant my time with my daughter would soon end. I could no longer walk with her, talk to her and get into bed with her every night like I had for the last few months.

I was in labour for around twelve hours, and it was painful – I cannot lie about that. I gave birth at home, so all I had was my mother's hand to hold. I could see she ached for me, but her being there meant that we both welcomed my daughter, her granddaughter, into this world. The blood that runs down your legs when giving birth is so warm and thick that you know it's blood without even looking down. That last big push when you must get the shoulders out – that is when you really feel it. I can still feel myself ripping and the blood running down, but you soon forget that as the legs and the rest come tumbling out. You forget until you go to the toilet, I should say. As we did not have anything to stitch my tear with, I had to just take care. I was lucky, and it was not as bad as others I have seen. My boss had the same experience of tearing, but she had doctors and weeks in bed to heal. For me, I had to be up and getting ready for the move. Peeing was like splintered glass passing between my legs at first. I cleaned myself with salty water and Dettol, but I was scared about how painful passing anything else would be. I ate little but, when the time came, it was as disgusting as it was painful. I could not strain or push hard, so it was months before I really emptied my system. I talked to my Mrs Boss about this because, when she had her baby, she was in bed for weeks. She has the best medical care in the country, and they even have these tablets to soften poo, so she tells me it passed like water, because she took too much. Her main issue was her husband, something she tells me I am lucky not to have. The idea of having sex again even years after giving birth is something that fills me with fear. It is very tight down there. I have had a feel and the way it all came back together I think is wrong, but it feels fine. All I need is somewhere to pee and have my period from. She needed hers for sex and to have another baby, so she is lucky to have had the medical help she did. But I don't think she had help with her fears, which is why she talks to me about it, I guess. I would have gone to my mum or my sister with my fears, but she does not have that, as her mum seems traditional and she does not have a sister.

Because of all this, she might not envy me, but I do not envy her either.

Looking after a rich woman's babies to support your own

If you want to see what a person is really like, look at how they treat the people working for them. To read about the nannies and maids working in the Middle East is to read a collection of horror stories. Beatings, sexual assault and even murder. One notorious case involved a young woman, Joanna Demafelis, being found frozen in her employers' fridge in 2018, more than a year after she was reported missing. Her Syrian employers are now under arrest. Those women 'lucky' enough to escape physical abuse are often paid very badly. One woman, explaining why she paid her nanny below minimum wage and gave her no time off, pointed out the woman had a 'very easy day and her own mobile phone'. To put a stop to these multiple abuses, the Filipino government has now demanded stricter contracts and better pay. This in turn has led to outraged employers in the Middle East bleating about how their would-be servants are demanding outrageous benefits, like a reasonable salary and time off.

I'm aware of how poverty can be romanticized, especially by those who have never experienced it, but after hearing Mia's story I was struck by the love she had for her family and the beauty of her village. I could also understand how, despite the wealth of her employer, Mia saw that this woman was in a gilded cage, her body a possession of her husband.

Marry

'The nurse told me not to get upset, it would just make it harder, but how could it be harder? I was losing my boy.'

I named him Adam. I'm not sure if it ...
I don't think it would be. I'm sure, just ...
ily, the family who adopted him wanted ...
me and how he came about. My baby was ...
he was perfect, with the bluest eyes I have ever ...
mother said my sin was that I was beautiful and s...
minded. You could say I was to be with a 'bastard' child
in the 80s, and not in the 60s. I've no idea why I use that
word, it's just what they called it. I was an unwed mother,
a teen pregnancy, a shamed girl. All these were said
about me, but of him it was just 'the condition'. Or I
could not keep a 'bastard', but he was not that. He was
wanted, he was loved and Sam, his father, wanted to
marry me. We had a plan, a plan that was summed up as
a teenage dream when we told my family. Sam's family
had a farm and we could go and live there with his parents. He would work on the farm and I would look after
the baby. This was a no-go; my mother would not have
me 'ruin' my life with a bastard baby and a deadbeat,
which she thought Sam was.

I was removed from school and basically locked up at
home for the next nine months. My father never spoke
to me and my bedroom became my cell. It was just Baby
and I in that room. Talking to your growing belly is not
something that you plan, but when you have no one else
to talk to you have little choice. I had no idea if it was
going to be a boy or a girl, but I kept our conversations
about the world. About school, what I enjoyed and what
I thought the baby would look like. Sam and I had blue

...he had darker hair, which made them pop. I drew pictures of what I thought the baby would look like and where I wished I could raise him or her. I was very slim before I got pregnant. I did cross-country and a million other sports. But being at home, I put on a lot of weight. I went from around eight stone to about eleven. The midwife had no idea that I was out of school and not allowed out, so she would tell me to ensure I was moving around a lot and to watch what I was eating. Food was the only comfort I had during my pregnancy. I was not allowed to speak to my friends, and most of them were not allowed to talk to me anyway. I was the whore who got knocked up. No one said it to my face, but even Sam stopped coming to the window when my parents went to sleep.

I used to eat whatever I could get my hands on, but chips were my favourite thing. I would sit there with loads of mayo and just eat and eat. It's odd, but I just wanted it to fill the emptiness, even though I had the baby growing inside, and I could feel it, there was also a cold emptiness. The warm chips would go right to that spot but not stick. It was only when my mum was told that I could be getting diabetes that she took notice. In her own way, giving me money for food was I think how she was telling herself it was okay, that what she was doing and how she was treating me was okay. She doubled the shopping of the things I would finish, which was everything.

When labour started, I screamed for Mum, and she was with me all the time. She held my hand, and I really thought that seeing me give birth might change things. I thought seeing me have the baby would remind her about having me, and maybe her love for me would come back. Even if that didn't happen, I thought she would see the baby and be unable to give it away. I was her first-born, just like this baby would be mine. Could she really let go of her first grandchild? It seemed she could. When my baby was born he didn't make a sound and my heart sank. I thought all the overeating and the crying meant that he did not make it. But in minutes he was screaming, and I looked to see if my mum had the look of relief I knew I had on her face, but there was nothing. She had started to look away again, her face grey, like it had been since I told her I was pregnant. My whole life has been grey since that day. It seemed to have rained every day since I found out. The night I had sex, which was just the once, I thought I was going to die. I really thought the Lord was going to strike me down. Sex before marriage in a wet shed was sinful beyond words. I did not die, but I got pregnant and it was nine months later that death in a living form would come to me. The child I carried and cried for would be taken away. The prayers that I said every night had gone unheard.

The next morning, when the nurse came, my mother was there. My father never came, and neither did Sam, but Mum never looked at Adam. She sat there looking at the wall as tears ran down my face, as everything was explained to me, not that I really took it in. She just sat there. The nurse told me not to get upset, it would just make it harder, but how could it be harder? I was losing my boy. I was losing the soul I had carried inside for nine long months and suffered with for two whole days. Leaving the hospital without him, I could not walk. I was weak from the labour, but I was also weak from the pain of losing him. The emptiness that I felt was not a gaping wound; it ached, it was bleeding and I knew in that moment nothing would ever fill it.

It's been twenty-eight years since my first pregnancy, my first child, and every day I think about him. For weeks my breasts leaked. That was the most physical pain post-labour that I felt. At times my breasts and my face would leak at the same time. I would cry and cry, then my breasts would follow. It made me think of him and if he was being fed at the same time.

I hoped, and I still pray, that he will come looking for me, but even if he does, he will just find someone who is struggling with so much. A few weeks later I turned sixteen and I could leave. I got a one-way ticket to Liverpool, and then Cardiff, where I have lived ever since. I still use food as my comfort, and it is the only thing I like. I don't use the term 'love', as the only things I loved I have lost. I've not spoken to my family for years. I have nothing to say to them. They took my life and soul away from me. Just because the idea of having a baby was something they placed in the box of marriage and what others thought.

I sometimes wonder if my baby was a girl and, with the world that we live in today, her getting pregnant, it being her first or tenth would not mean losing her whole life. The world is just a different place.

I just hope that if my son ever gets someone pregnant

he stands by her and that, even if it doesn't work out, he supports the mother of his child.

Forced adoption

If Marry's family had supported her, they could have ridden out the gossip and made Adam a proud part of their family. As Marry said herself, this was the 80s. Instead, like millions of other families, they chose to shame their daughter and force her to give up her baby. Nobody told her she could keep Adam – not her mother, nor the nurse or her father. And why didn't anyone from the adoption agency point out this inconvenient fact? Could it be they had a vested interest in taking a lovely new baby boy from a young, traumatized girl who had no idea of her rights and wouldn't make a fuss? The pain and suffering caused by the twisted idea of being 'respectable' has recently been raised in the Irish Parliament. The Irish Taoiseach, Leo Varadkar, apologized in June 2018 for a spate of illegal adoptions carried out in Ireland up until 1969. This apology followed one made five years previously about the appalling Magdalene Laundries, ostensibly for 'fallen women' but really a means to get rid of troublesome girls. Adam's adoption wasn't illegal but still caused Marry a lifetime of anguish. The recent overwhelming repeal of the Eighth Amendment shows that attitudes are changing, but too late for Marry.

Not at all ironically, the countries where legal abortion is most severely restricted tend also to have the poorest maternal and baby care. Anti-choice activists trumpet what they call a 'culture of life', but what this means is no sex before heterosexual marriage, no contraception and shaming single girls who get pregnant.

Kris

'They should have given me an episiotomy, but
they said tearing is "natural" and heals better,
that it allows your body to work how it should.
Cutting me would be very medical and harder
to heal. Maybe a small tear, but not when
your vagina feels like it's crashed through a
windscreen.'

Not that I ever had one, but the birth of my first son put an end to my porn career. He came out with his arms sideways, like he was yawning with his arms stretched out, and it tore me apart.

The medical lingo is a 'third-degree laceration'. It means the tear goes from the vaginal muscle through the perineal skin and muscle. In real terms, I was so badly ripped up I was kept in hospital for a week, which is unheard of in London. Usually, they're ready to kick you out as soon as the afterbirth squelches out. I was drugged up, so I didn't feel any real pain, but I could still feel a distant throb. They should have given me an episiotomy, but they said tearing is 'natural' and heals better, that it allows your body to work how it should. Cutting me would be very medical and harder to heal. Maybe a small tear, but not when your vagina feels like it's crashed through a windscreen. Anyway, there is nothing 'natural' about my body now. I'm like Frankenstein's monster between my legs – all I need are the bolts, and it aches physically as much as it does emotionally.

I've had two operations to help make simple actions like sitting down more comfortable, but it's going to be a long road and I'm still not sure if I'll ever be back to normal. My son is almost one now and, for the last few months, I've been unable to pick him up. I just can't get down on the ground. Even *thinking* about it is painful. Bending down is no more – I'm like an old woman who can't sit on the floor.

I make light of it when I talk to my boyfriend, and he is supportive, but he's not in the bathroom with me or being examined on the cold bed in the clinic. He wasn't there when I first took a mirror into the bathroom with me. He wasn't there when that horrific image hit me. I know it was only a few weeks after my first operation and the stitches were new and raw, but I almost passed out. I was never one to look at my lady parts as somewhere to put on show, but I was familiar with them. I first looked at her when I was thirteen and got my first few hairs. I like that you give her a name – Asha – and see her as a sister. Maybe I might do that. Maybe it will help me reconnect. When I first saw my pussy . . . I think I'll use that word to call it . . . everything else seems too medical or offensive and I'm bored of my pussy being either of those things.

When I saw her she was odd. My skin is dark, very

dark, but I was pink between my legs. My lips, just like the ones on my face, were pink with a brown strip. Soon I was covered in hair and it was in my later teens I got into shaving then waxing. I experimented when I was in uni, so I must have seen other girls' pussies. Is that what you call more than one? They were all different but beautiful, so beautiful. If I could get back to how I was, trust me, I wouldn't complain about it at all. I would love my pussy and never say a bad word about it. Maybe I should call her *minou*, the French for 'pussy'.

I want to have another baby, but that means I'll have to wait for real constructive surgery to be done. I will have to live like this, knowing what I look like down there, feeling sick and acting like it's all fine. No one tells you about these things, they don't warn you that it might go wrong. That you will hold your baby in your arms and wonder how you will manage when you can't even sit up, when pissing is stinging pain. When you can feel stitches sticking out like wire, when you wipe yourself and must wipe so carefully, because getting anything into the places that aren't healed is something you really don't want to do. Getting an infection is so painful, it's thrush on acid, the pain, aching and itching . . . oh my God, *the itching*. You itch like mad and, because you can't help scratching, you end up getting raw. But I now take so much care I could clear a murder scene. It was like a crime scene, the first few weeks, with blood everywhere, and sometimes it would clot, so I would have to sit in salty warm water to loosen it all up. I could sit in the bath for ten minutes and the water resembled red wine.

There was also a lot of bush after a few weeks. I waxed just before having the baby, but it all came back and that didn't help. After a while I could just use scissors to trim the sides, it was that long.

It's really been hard, and it hurts in so many ways, but I haven't cried about it, mainly because I don't know what I'd be crying for. Is it for the body I've lost, the time with my child, the relationship I had with my boyfriend that I would be crying for? I think I'm mostly just fed up. Of the self-hate, the 'How is it down there today?' from the doctor, the nurse, my mum, and soon the milkman, when he reads this. I'm not ashamed – I'm just lost. Have I said that before? I am honestly so lost. I don't know what I want but I know I must be a mum. I must raise this ball of cells, now a human, take care of him. I must go back to work and be professional. I have a home, friends and family to care for. I guess I must get back to all that and keep this all under wraps. Under wraps, that is, until I can unwrap a new pussy.

Birth injuries

As Kris says, nobody ever tells you about these things when you're pregnant – 'things' being the possibility of birth injuries. It's part of this natural schtick we hear about pregnancy and babies. Funny how nobody ever suggests a return to natural dentistry, though.

In 2008, a Mumsnet user called Cyee started a thread for women who had suffered birth injuries such as severe tearing. 'In my own experience, this whole area is a bit taboo,' she wrote. 'In fact, the consultants reckon there are many women who have some symptoms related to the above who never seek treatment. The thought of women embarrassed to discuss these matters is awful, yet that seems to be the case.' From the enormous response and continuation of the thread, there appear to be many women in a similar situation to Kris, suffering from painful and itchy scar tissue, distress over incontinence and, perhaps worst of all, multiple examples of indifference from the medical profession. And yet it's estimated that over 20,000 women a year in the UK suffer silently from PTSD, a condition usually associated with soldiers and violent crime, but in this case following birth trauma.

Ivory

'We are experiencing so many firsts, and our
first pregnancy also means we can have lots of
sex for the next few months without periods.'

When I first found out I was pregnant, I had that *how the hell did that happen?* face. Well, I do know how, of course. I was married, and we did 'fox'. I still can't say the word 'sex'. I'm trapped between being a teen and my mother when it comes to the situation I'm in.

Does that sound stupid? To me, marriage and babies go hand in hand. I remember you saying you were only okay with a baby that came from the man who you loved. I'm not sure if I love my husband like we talked about and I certainly didn't think a baby would be in the mix so soon.

But I do want this baby and I hope when he or she is born it's all I hope for. I hope I'm not mistaking my excitement for being scared, and this is something I really want. I'm not completely sure and only my faith in God is what's keeping me going. My biggest question is, have I made a mistake? Will this baby hold back my career? Will I be as carefree as I was a few weeks ago, before I found out?

When we booked into the clinic to see the midwife I was nervous. I wanted her to tell me I was wrong about being pregnant, and I was too young, and it was too early in my marriage. But I was pregnant, and it was all real. The next thing we – I say 'we', but what *I* had to do was tell my mum. It was so embarrassing!

Till then, everyone is just assuming you're having sex but there is no proof till you're knocked up. We got knocked up within five weeks! What would the people at work say? What would my non-Somali friends say? And what the hell would you say? No, I knew what you would say. 'That was quick!' and then ask if I was happy. That was one of the questions that still knocks about in my head. *Am* I happy? Honestly, it feels so odd, this thing growing inside me, married to a man I don't really know but placing my faith in God that he is the one.

My faith, how I got married and why, is something not many understand. Maybe fear drove me. I was almost thirty, everyone was married, and I do believe that it's part of your faith. I'll be a mother before I've been married or known the man I'm married *to* for a year. I'm shopping for babygros with a man I'm only just getting to know, and this seems an odd way of doing things, but so far it seems to be working. We are experiencing so many firsts, and our first pregnancy also means we can have lots of sex for the next few months without periods.

I say that because the sex is amazing, and the idea of stopping when I have the baby is beyond scary. I'm not sure how I waited thirty years to have it. Maybe I was so on heat I got knocked up quickly, but sex is so, so good. At first, of course, I was scared and nervous. We did not kiss till the night of our wedding and, Lord, I prayed it would be good. I got my 'pink book' with all the Islamic do's and don'ts. I was waxed and ready, like a chicken ready for the roasting. Oh my God, not that footballer kind of roasting. For a holy person, I am coming out with lots of unholy shit.

I'm thinking that I got pregnant on the first night. He wanted to talk and make me feel at ease, but after ten minutes of niceties, I just wanted to jump him. Something just came over me, he was like that first bite after fasting all day. And I had been fasting for a long time. It was a little painful and I didn't really know what I was doing, but only that I liked kissing him and couldn't stop myself.

We didn't stop after that! The pregnancy, I think, has made me hornier – although he does seem to have issues in satisfying my needs. I'm not sure if I will be this forward after the baby is born or if I will even be able to *have*, let alone *want*, sex when I get bigger.

It'll be odd, that I will have no idea what sex is like before being pregnant, apart from the first few times I had sex. My boobs are bigger, they feel better when touched – or maybe they just like being touched. I've no idea, really. I'm in the mood for sex all the time. I'm not sure if that's because I'm with child or because I'm a horny so-and-so.

I won't kid you. I'm worried about what down there will feel like after the baby, as my husband isn't small, so I'm praying that will be okay. Faith and fucking seem to be the story of my life right now.

Sex in pregnancy

There are several reasons why women can enjoy great sex in pregnancy. The first being, of course, that you can't get pregnant, which can be amazingly freeing. Secondly, you can have as much as 50 per cent more blood flowing through you, meaning your vulva becomes engorged more easily, which can also increase the intensity of your orgasm. Thirdly, extra oestrogen and progesterone flying round your body can also make your breasts more sensitive. So, if you're in a relationship and your partner can get past the 'precious vessel' idea, you can have great sex together, or alone, if he or she can't keep up.

Make the most of it, though, because lots of women say that, after they give birth, sex is off the menu for quite a while. Why? Well, depending on the kind of birth you have, your vagina could either feel a bit sore or as though someone has put a live hand grenade down your knickers. Even though your breasts might look enormously inviting, they're also engorged and, again, many women don't want their partner anywhere near them if the baby has been suckling every two seconds. And finally, with a tiny human who needs your undivided attention, women often report they want their body back. And by this I don't mean 'back in their size-ten jeans' but their body, alone and not being touched, stroked or generally felt up. As one woman said, 'I gave him a child. The least he can do is go jerk off in the shower.'

Hibo

'The nurse knew that I could not go home
without having the termination. They were so
kind, so understanding, I don't remember it
being painful, I remember seeing the nurse
looking down at me, holding my hand.'

I have been pregnant four times, but no one apart from my social worker and the doctors I saw know about my first one. I was eighteen, so I was not really that young and should have known better, but I was so in love and I trusted him. I had moved from Holland to London with my family when I was eleven, and it was hard to settle in. There I was, a Dutch Somali girl, and now living in London. I could not find my place in this world, so I was what you could call a loner. I met the father of the baby at a coffee shop I was working at after college. He was tall, handsome and Somali, so when he asked me out I was taken aback. I am not sure if it is possible for me to blush, but I did, and I was so nervous when we first met for a coffee. He was lovely and said he had seen me around for a while but thought maybe I was taken. Yeah, me, taken, right. *Whatever* is what I thought, but I said nothing. I must have looked like a total idiot just sitting there, but I was so shocked he was interested in me. I was not cool, and I was far from hot. But he seemed into me and it was nice that after the coffee he asked me to the movies. He was respectful and knew that I did not believe in sex before marriage. He accepted this and was shocked when I told him he was the first person I had ever kissed. The more I came to know him, the more I fell for him. He said that being eighteen and from a community where dating is not the done thing, he had to try everything. This meant that no one knew we were dating. I would overhear other girls talking about him and how they were going to make a move on him. These were girls I could only dream of ever being. I think that this and the fact that, yes, I fancied him, were at the root of why I changed my mind about sex before marriage. We had been together for six months when we had sex. It was in a flat his cousin shared with someone else, a disgusting, messy place that smelled like a locker room. After we had sex it all changed. I could not stop crying and he did not even want to hold me or tell me it was going to be okay. It was so cold in that room, and so was he after he dropped me off that evening. I did not text him that night, as I had no idea what to say, and he did not text either.

Days before we had sex he was telling me I was the most beautiful girl in the world, and how he could not wait to spend the rest of his life with me. I tell myself now as I tell this story and have been for a few years that maybe he felt guilty and that is why he did what he did. When I tried to call him a few days after we had sex the phone kept cutting off. I texted him, thinking that maybe he was in a bad network area, but nothing. When I tried to look him up on Facebook, he was gone. We were not friends, as I did not want anyone seeing we were connected, but I could always see him, and he was not that limited, so I could see where he was tagged and who he was hanging with.

But now nothing, he was gone; I had been blocked. At first, I did not know this, but I used my sister's phone to look him up and there he was. The same grin I would look at, now filling me with fear and distress, not excitement and happiness. He had cut me off. He had cut me off after taking the most precious thing to me in that moment.

My heart and soul were broken. I hated myself so much. I told myself I was smarter than this. How could this be? What would become of me? Would he be telling all his mates about me now, slut-shaming me, making sure I would never be kissed or loved again? I stayed in bed for weeks, crying and wanting to die. I could not talk to anyone. I did not really have any friends, and my family would kill me, my sister would hate me and my mother would disown me. I had no one, but the heartache was not the worst. I knew I had missed a period, but that was normal, I did not have one every month and, during my GCSEs, the stress meant that I missed a few months. I thought that was it, but after three months I got worried. I also needed a note from the doctor because I had missed so many weeks of university I was about to be kicked out. As soon as I walked in I just broke down crying. This GP I had seen once when I needed a flu jab seemed to be the only person I could speak to. Everything just came flooding out and, without a word, she came out from behind her desk and sat next to me. I will never forget her voice when she held my hand and said, 'I would like us to do a pregnancy test, just to see where we stand.' Those words stopped my world. I knew instantly both what the result would be and what I had to do. I could not even tell my family about having a boyfriend. I could not have a baby. I did not want one. I could not have one. I could not.

Taking the test, I was shaking. I could not pee; my body went into shutdown. I drank more water, I ran the tap, but nothing for an hour. My head just did not want to know what my heart and body knew. Walking back to the doctor's room was just a minute, but it felt like a lifetime, and waiting for the five minutes for the test to complete was several lifetimes. I kept saying, 'I don't want it . . . I don't want it,' but it was not that simple. I was eighteen weeks by the time it was confirmed, and

I had no idea why I was not showing, but I guess you don't. Walking home, I was so scared that it would be written all over my face and that someone would work it out. My family would find out and I would be done for. Really done for. My family is not liberal, my family would kill me, they really would, or I would kill myself if they found out. I had told the doctor this, and that I was happy to have an abortion there and then, but it seems that is not how it worked. She was worried that I was not mentally ready, and I had not taken it in. Of course I was mentally unwell. I had been in bed for weeks, crying and barely eating. I had only washed occasionally, and my hair was in knots.

I had three appointments before I was booked in for the abortion. I was also appointed a social worker. I was eighteen, almost nineteen, but my mental health was not good and, rightly, they were worried about me doing something stupid. When the date came I could not move. The social worker knew and was waiting for me around the corner. When everyone left I called her, and she came to my house to basically help me out of bed.

I was so scared and, when I saw the clamp on the table, I broke down. The nurse knew that I could not go home without having the termination. They were so kind, so understanding. I don't remember it being painful, I remember seeing the nurse looking down at me, holding my hand. The doctor did not look at me; he was African, I remember that. My legs were shaking, and they had to help me down after I was asleep as I could not move. Have you ever been so scared that you just lose control and are dead cold? That's what I was. In the scan to date the pregnancy I saw it move, and I still see it. That is what I kept thinking about when I woke up. I wanted to know what it looked like, what they did with it, what would happen to me. Would I be going to hell? Would I be able to forgive myself? Would people find out? Neither the nurse, the GP nor the social worker would answer these questions.

For weeks I wished every night that I would never wake up, but with months of counselling this soon changed. I started to get back to school, seeing people again. I started taking care and pride in what I looked like. It was a long process. I moved out of London for uni and I just boxed up that whole experience in my head.

That was ten years ago, and I cannot say I totally forgot about it, but it would be days, sometimes weeks, before it came into my mind. Then about two years ago I met my husband when I came back to London. He is also Somali, and he is a great man. He was the first man I trusted and allowed into my life after what happened to me. I met him at a lecture and, as he was religious, there was no issue about no sex before marriage – not that I would do that again. I have been praying for forgiveness since I lost my virginity, so the idea of men and sex was something I could live without. The closer I got to thirty, my family started to talk, and I gave in. They would give my number to a few people and I would talk to them. It would be the usual 'How are you, and are you interested in meeting for coffee?' I would meet up, and then nothing. I did not really care; it would mean my mum was off my back for a few weeks.

When I met my husband I was not interested, but his kindness won me over. He seemed down to earth and really interested in me. I thought he could be the one who would heal me, and I needed the love that I could feel from him. When I accepted his proposal I thought that chapter in my life was over. I hoped that I would never have to think about it, let alone tell him.

It was all going well and when we found out we were pregnant he was over the moon. I was uneasy, though. At first, I could not really feel any connection with this pregnancy, and then suddenly the pain of all I had tried to forget came rushing back. I pushed it all away; it was going to be okay, he was not going to leave me, we were married, I told myself. But the pain was not fear – it was guilt and, just before twenty-three weeks, just around the same time as I had got rid of my first pregnancy, I miscarried. This time, I got to see the baby. It was a girl, she was so beautiful, so tiny. In that moment I knew it was God telling me something. I could not handle it. I looked at my husband and I just wanted to tell him. But I could not. He had just lost a child and I did not want to add to that with the loss of a wife he thought he knew. We have not been able to get pregnant again, and I don't think I want to. I don't think I can mentally take it. I know I need help again, but I also just wanted to tell someone this. I need someone that looks like me to talk to and tell me it is okay and that it will all be okay.

I am physically well and feel it, but mentally not there yet.

Stillbirth

A pregnancy loss is a miscarriage up to twenty-four weeks. After that, it's a stillbirth. Hibo suffered the agonizing loss of her baby at twenty-three weeks, and she's right – she needs to talk to someone who can reassure her that she was just unlucky and having the abortion didn't *cause* the stillbirth, any more than being gay causes hurricanes.

Giving birth to a stillborn baby is horrific, but with good medical care and gentle guidance it can be survivable. Many women can't bear the idea of seeing their dead newborn, but midwives will often gently suggest they reconsider, as dressing the baby, taking photos and holding him or her can instigate the healing process. As one woman said, 'My daughter might not be alive, but she was still my daughter.'

Fia

'You are the only person who has asked how
I was, and not "Are you okay?"'

I moved to Canada when I was twelve with my uncle and brother. I am the only girl in my family and before I left I promised my mum I would be good and, because I was twelve, I meant it. I was good at school and held it together. I never showed how much I missed my mum and how being in a house with two men was, and still is, odd. I was lucky that, within months, another family from the same village as me moved in down the road. They adopted me, we got close, and their mum began to fill the hole created by my mum being so far away. I got so close that I ended up marrying one of the boys. He was the first person I ever kissed or slept with, and then he became my home. I was seventeen when he told me he liked me. I can't say it was news to me, as he was the youngest and shyest of the three boys. When we went to parties he would be the one driving, as he didn't drink. He's also very smart. So, I agreed to go to a movie and dinner with him. We dated for a few weeks before he even tried to make a move, and when we finally went to bed together he was so gentle, really caring. I wasn't nervous, but I wasn't that excited either, and it was over very soon. We had to be quiet, because we were in his bedroom and the idea of anyone hearing would be a nightmare. His family, as open as they were to dating, are still African and trad-itional. Sex before marriage was a no-no. I can't say I remember much of it. It wasn't painful the first time, and the next time we went away to a cheap, smelly motel, but we needed to be alone and that's all we had money for. This time he wasn't so gentle, and it did hurt. I asked him to stop at one point, but he just kept going. It would have been okay if we hadn't forgotten to use protection as well. I tried to get the morning-after pill, but the place near us was run by someone who knew me and my family, and I thought they would tell everyone, which I am sure they would have. I kept my fingers crossed and hoped beyond hope that it would be okay.

I should have kept my legs crossed, as keeping my fingers crossed didn't work. When I found out I was pregnant I wanted to call my mum or my auntie back home, but I knew they would be so disappointed in me. When I told him, I thought I would be in tears, but there were none and I found strength somewhere. Deep down, I was hoping that he would suggest an abortion, because he was off to college soon and had life planned out. I was still in high school and wanted to travel after I finished. I wanted to go home, I wanted to visit my mum, I wanted so much more. When we told his family there was even less understanding. His mother cried and had a literal fit on the kitchen floor. She called me every name under the sun and screamed at whatever god had brought me into their house. I get it, I suppose. This was her youngest and brightest son, and now, instead of building her a mansion in Africa and showering her with gold, he was going to be a dad and would have to get married. That was never going to happen anyway, but it was her dream and I was this whore coming to take it all away. I got it: I'd seen this scenario played out on TV. I don't know if it was just an extreme example of African mothers that she fitted to a T. I had never got those parodies, I had never known them to be true or not. Sorry – I keep going on about me being this *Oliver*-like child, the orphan who wanted more, but that's what it felt like, and there's nothing lonelier than having a mother out there but not being able to see her.

I felt so empty that it made me sick just thinking about it. Thank you for asking me how I am. You are the only person who has asked how I was, and not 'Are you okay?'

It was decided that we would get married right away and say the baby was conceived on the wedding night. Yes, that old story. From Africa to America, we have all heard of those wedding-night babies, born a month or two early but somehow looking overdue. No, it's okay to giggle. It was so fucking stupid. He agreed, he loved me, and maybe I should be grateful for that, but it's hard to be grateful when you feel so hopeless. It was also decided he should go to his chosen college, which was out of state. Meanwhile, I would stay and live with his mum. Lucky me.

I sound ungrateful, but his mum didn't see me as the one for her son, and living under the same roof was going to be hard. How hard, I had no idea, because four weeks after Sam left I woke up in the middle of the night with the sharpest pain I've ever felt in my life. It was so painful that at one point I think I jumped right out of bed. If I was a cat, I would have been on the ceiling. I had no idea what it was till I went to the toilet and saw the blood on my knickers. It was not bright, it was dark and thick; it was warm, but my body was cold. It was late and the whole house was asleep and, knowing my new mother-in-law hated me, getting her up was the last thing on my mind. I don't know how long I sat on that toilet and hoped for the blood to stop, but it kept oozing out. The back pain was so intense that I couldn't stand. I was so alone and the only person I could think of calling was my brother, but I couldn't bring myself to do it. I ended up calling my brother-in-law, and he still had a key so could get into the house. My feet gave way when I tried to stagger to the door to meet him. By the time he got to me I was in a pool of blood. My mother-in-law talks about it as if it were a massacre. He had woken her when he walked into the bathroom to see me lying there. He joked that he was whiter than I was, which I'm not even sure is possible. I needed several litres of blood and it was a few days before I could even talk, let alone stand up.

My husband rushed to my side and, because I was out of it for so long, I didn't have time to think about what had happened as the pain was too much. But when I came out of hospital I didn't really know what I felt. I was sad – I still am – but I couldn't feel anything or express much for a while. If you ask how I am, you allow me to tell you what I am feeling, which is a lot, from aching physically, emotionally, to feeling empty and confused.

My husband has never asked, and it's now been years and things have changed between us.

After I came out of the hospital he left a week later and the attention or even interest in me or asking if I was 'okay' stopped. When he came to visit we slept in the same bed, but nothing happened. He was such a sweet soul, even if he lacked skills in bed, and that early time still sticks out. Now there is nothing. I have initiated the few times we've had sex. It's not as rough, but there is no love or kindness from him. I have no idea where that all went. My heart was broken in so many places. I am married to a man who doesn't really know how he feels, I've lost a baby I'm not sure I wanted, I'm so far from a mother I'm not sure if I really miss the baby. I'm not ashamed to say I was depressed till I took a trip away from the US, and till I started to distance myself from him and his family. I'm now seeking to find my own path and the idea of what my life could and should be. The pregnancy took me on a path I never expected. They say childbirth is painful, but so is a fucking miscarriage. Giving birth, you take something home, but with a miscarriage you leave empty-handed, but with all this grief and confusion you can't see, feelings you must work through, rather than just learning how to change a nappy.

Miscarriage

Misha miscarried at thirteen weeks. 'I'd felt this growling pain in my stomach all morning. I stood up and felt something break inside me – my waters, probably. Then this gush of bright red oxygenated blood just poured out. There was so much of it.' She remembers sitting on the toilet as the blood ran, while her partner held her hand and kept flushing. 'Don't look,' he said. They went to the Early Pregnancy Unit the next day, and Misha remembers being sat next to a woman who was quietly jubilant over an IVF twin pregnancy. 'She asked me how far along I was, and big, snotty tears just rolled down my face,' says Misha. 'It would be nice if a miscarrying woman could sit in a different room from a pregnant one.' When she and her partner went into a room for her ultrasound, Misha noticed a strategic box of tissues next to the couch, and a pile of leaflets. Then the agonizing silence as the nurse gently moved the probe and searched the empty screen. 'I'm sorry, but the products of conception have left the womb,' she said. 'I'll never forget those words,' said Misha. 'It sounded as though they'd gone for a walk. *Products* of conception? My partner was picking up the leaflets and talking to the nurse. It's so hard for men, they're expected to be strong, but there's nothing physical for them to mourn. The foetus is just a bundle of cells – they don't carry it or have that emotional connection. But they have to cope with their partner in terrible pain.'

Because there were no clear medical reasons for the miscarriage, Misha, like a lot of women, turned to self-blame. 'I flayed myself about every cup of coffee or the glass of wine I'd had before I knew I was pregnant. I talked to my GP, who said that miscarriage is the poor relation of infertility. That women find out they are pregnant far earlier than they used to, and because there isn't a great deal of research into miscarriages, women (surprise) blame themselves.' The Miscarriage Association says there are no 'shoulds', but many women do feel guilty or embarrassed about mourning an early loss and quietly swallow their grief. A *Woman's Hour* phone-in on miscarriage had women of sixty and seventy crying because they hadn't felt they could properly mourn at the time.

'I was lucky,' says Misha. 'Nobody in my family said

anything crass about how there must have been something wrong with it, although there probably was. I was just left with the overriding feeling that, overnight, my body had turned from a tender incubator into a briskly efficient disposal unit.'

Faz

'I think they are ashamed of people tweeting
dead babies, or maybe they cared about women
in need, like I was.'

I'm going to London because that's where our life is. I hoped I would have had the baby there but, as you can see, he's here with me in this camp. I came to the Jungle when I was five months pregnant, and it was cold and dirty and I cried for hours because we paid so much money for a smuggler to take us to London and now we are here. I call him that now because I know now that's what he was, but we trusted him and thought he would do right by us. My husband keeps telling me it won't be much longer, but the baby is not four months, it will be cold again soon, and I will be marking a year here. I married my husband because I wanted to get out of Afghanistan and he had a plan. He has family in London and that's why we will not and cannot stay in France. There's nothing and no connections for people like us. Afghanistan and its people are old news, we are the subject of posters and political debates, we are in the shadows here in the West and back home, and I want a future.

I had no idea I was pregnant when we left. Had I known, I would have still come, but only because I wouldn't have told him. He would have left me behind and then there would be no way I would get to London.

I know where London is. My in-laws live in Wood Green. I don't know where that is. There are no hospitals where I am from in Afghanistan, but there is family and kindness. The women in France have been nice, but not understanding each other was hard. Have you been scared and unable to communicate your fear? That was the worst, the not knowing what was going on. When it is your first, you don't know much, but people give you hints. My mother would talk to her sister about her own births when she was pregnant, and the same with my sister-in-law.

I had nothing, and I just made it all up. It is not hard to have a baby – they just come out the way they were created – but it's just horrible not knowing if you are doing it right. It is embarrassing and puts you under a lot of stress, with all these people looking at you, saying something you cannot understand, making faces. I now know they were telling me when to breathe and push. As I didn't understand, I just pushed hard when I needed to. That was a mistake, and a painful one. When you have drugs, you can tear, but you don't feel it right away. The only time I was treated like a human in this whole process was when I was giving birth, even if I did not feel it.

You are given access to leave the camp and go to the hospital. I think they are ashamed of people tweeting dead babies, or maybe they cared about women in need, like I was.

It's hard to stop when something is forcing its way out. In my house back in Afghanistan we had one toilet, and I remember when I was a kid my father and brother would always go first if they needed to go. My father used to take what seemed like hours. I needed to have a shit urgently once, but I had to wait, and it was so painful holding it in when it was coming out, and it was really coming out. It took all I had to hold it in, and it was too late to go anywhere else. That was the last time I had to hold anything in when your body wanted it out. This was a million times worse and there was no mind over matter. I can talk about this now because there are a few women here who have or had children. Some of them had to leave them wherever they are from. Now I know I should have pushed when they wanted me to, but I didn't understand them all shouting and mouthing at me and making gestures. It's lonely not understanding someone trying to help you. I was so scared. It wasn't a question of fearing death, as I almost died several times in my life, many of those on the way to this hell hole.

The real pain has been since having the baby. I only knew I was in labour when my waters broke. I was in labour for hours, it seemed, but it was not that agonizing. It was certainly painful, but I was expecting something that would bring me to my knees. The pain was just a level up from period pain. It was around my back, and my belly was tightening up, but I just thought that it was the baby moving. When you are sleeping somewhere held together with string and basically on the floor for weeks while heavily pregnant, everything is uncomfortable. My back had been aching for months, my feet were always cold – walking in mud and sleeping on the floor will do that to you, so when the labour started I was too cold and achy already to know.

There was no screaming. I had nothing to scream about. I am blessed in as much as I had hoped to be having my first child in Europe, with a home to go back to. I also prayed I did not give birth or miscarry on the way to the Jungle. I saw women give birth in the middle of nowhere, and there were no doctors or anyone to help them. They would just get back up the next day and keep walking. When the war was in full swing and bombs were dropping my sister-in-law told me about a woman who gave birth in a shelter, with children and men around. I am not sure if that was true, but I am also not sure how people could have sex when there is a war going on.

Because I ripped badly, I can say that the pain has been when I sit, something which I do a lot because there is not much you can do in the camp. I am not planning on having sex while we are here, so that is lucky, for me. I know my husband would want to have another baby right away, as we have had a daughter. He wants a boy, and he is not holding back because he cares about me or how I feel, it is because it is easy to see into our house and you can hear everything. I am unable to change if he is not here to hold up the thick blankets. I have no idea who he thinks will get off on seeing a woman with bloody underwear and a belly, but there is never much sense to what men believe.

It's hard trying to keep myself from getting an infection. I have been using warm water and salt every time I pass urine, and when I do a shit I have to use my hands to get it out. It is too painful to push too hard. I must put my hands against my downstairs and help it pass rather than just pushing. I don't go often and sometimes I pour warm salty water as I pass what I need to. It soothes the pain and keeps the area clean. I have been told by the nurse of the site that it's working, and I am not as raw as I was a few weeks ago. There is nothing they can really do; the conditions are how they are.

I will be sitting here waiting, with my sore bottom and my big, red, wet boobs.

Giving birth in a refugee camp

Help Refugees is a grassroots organization dedicated to improving the lives of refugees. They aim to provide both emergency help, and for long-term need, and are currently running projects all over Europe, including Greece, France, Italy, Serbia, and in Iraq and the Lebanon – wherever there are refugee camps. The latest addition are camps in Rakhine, where there's been a recent spike in births due to rape by Myanmar militia.

In refugee camps, as Faz discovered, care in pregnancy

is practically zero, but as Dr Nikitis Kanakis of Doctors of the World pointed out, 'A lot of people talk about the cost of medical care in Europe. They forget that *not* giving care has a cost. Antenatal care costs much less than giving birth to a handicapped child.'

Baby Jacob

'For the first time in my life I had no idea what was going to happen, but I felt that I had power over my life.'

He was the most beautiful thing, and I fell in love with him as soon as I saw him. I'd never held a baby before him and he was just perfect. Well, to me he was, but I could see in my husband's face that he didn't agree. We had been told during our twelve-week scan that something was wrong. It was a terrible shock to us. I'd met my husband at uni and we had planned everything. I was a stylist and he was a lawyer. We had moved to London, had amazing friends, a home we loved, and it was now the right time to have a baby. It was all meant to be so simple: get married, buy a house, then have a baby. So, when we were told there was something wrong, our world fell apart. I didn't want to believe it, or even think about it. I left the appointment not having heard what the doctor had said. He had read out a list – our baby had a series of complex medical problems. There was nothing they could do. My husband and I couldn't take any of it in. We drove home in silence. That evening we had tickets to see *Wicked* with some of our friends and their children. I didn't want to cancel as I refused to believe what was happening. Tom, being American, wanted to talk, but I just didn't have the words or the strength to speak them. We went to see the show and escaped from all that I knew we would have to deal with when we got home.

The next morning, reality hit. I got up at 5 a.m., attempting to get ready for work. Tom would normally go for a run, but he was still in bed. It's odd thinking about it. When there is something wrong with a baby in utero, everyone assumes you try to forget about that pregnancy, but everything that led up to Jacob's birth is my first pregnancy and has shaped who I am today as a mother and as a woman. I walked naked into the bathroom and saw my belly. In that moment I knew all that I'd planned and wished for was gone. Tears rolled down my face. I had no idea why I was crying, but I did know it wasn't about being pregnant.

Tom and I had made this baby after watching Mo Farah win gold at London 2012. We had been so excited after we found out and we wanted the baby so much. None of that had changed for me.

I walked back out of the bathroom, woke Tom up and told him that, no matter what, I wanted this baby and we were going to work it all out. Fucking hell, I cannot believe I am about to tell you and the world this, but what happened next ripped my heart out. With bloodshot eyes, Tom stared at me and said, 'God, I knew this was going to happen.' I'd no idea what he was talking about, but he sat up and reminded me about a conversation we'd had years ago. 'You know how I feel. I don't want to bring a child into this world that's going to suffer. Hun, you know this, and we talked about it.'

We had talked about it, yes, but just that. But there's a big difference between an abstract conversation about something that hadn't even happened at that point and the reality of Tom rejecting our baby because it wasn't what we expected. All I could say was 'Are you kidding me?' But he wasn't. We sat in bed, talked and cried for hours, but neither of us was going to change our mind.

We decided that we needed more information about Jacob's condition. I jumped on the internet as Tom went to talk to the doctor and set up an appointment. I had no idea what I was looking for, I hadn't listened to what the doctor had said at the scan, or if he had even given us a name for what was wrong with our baby. It sounds mad now, but I found myself googling 'can a scan be wrong?' and 'scan mistakes'. I hunted for anything that would confirm my belief that the doctor was wrong and our baby was as perfect as everything else in our life.

I use the word 'perfect' because at the back of my mind was the worry of what people would say if I broke down and asked, *Why us?* It's really one of the things I've never said out loud, but *Why us?* was the main question I asked myself, but never said out loud. And especially not to Tom, as I was the one fighting for Jacob.

We got an appointment the next day, and the doctor told us that we were 'lucky' to find out so early. Since that day, I can't bear to hear that word. Yes, I was so 'lucky' that my world was falling apart. Jacob had several complications and we were told that, even if he was born, he wouldn't live long and, if he was 'lucky', maybe he would make it to the age of one.

Walking out of the hospital, I felt the life I knew slipping, but looking back, something else took over. For the first time in my life I had no idea what was going to happen, but I felt that I had power over my life. That sounds bloody odd, but my life has always been planned out. I was going to go to Oxford, I knew I was going to live in London and one day meet a handsome man. That's where the idea of 'perfect' comes in – my life was always well ordered and planned, but I don't think I had any control over that. My mother was a socialite, and my father a banker. I went to the best schools, travelled, and boys were never an issue. I just went with it, got the grades, loved the sports I was meant to love and partied with my friends. When Tom came along we dated for a year, had the engagement, and then the big wedding in the country estate, followed by the house in a lovely green part of London. But throughout this 'perfect' life I never stopped and asked if this was what I really wanted or if I should try something else, or just explored a few other ways of living. I'm not even sure if I knew what else was out there.

But in deciding to carry on with the pregnancy, scared as I was, with no idea what was ahead, I had never felt so much in control. Tom made it clear that he thought it was a mistake and that he needed time to think, so I went to my parents for the weekend. They agreed with

Tom and wanted me to 'think', even though I'd been doing nothing but thinking for weeks. They talked about how my life would never be the same and questioned my ability to cope. But my mind was made up. I was continuing this pregnancy, whatever the results. I started looking online for support groups. Tom never came, nor did he ask about them. He and my parents just hoped I would change my mind and go back to being the more compliant Beth they knew.

His mother was the only person who supported me, but that was mainly because she was religious and, as sweet as she was, Bible verses were not what I needed.

The night I went into labour I was still holding out hope that all the doctors were wrong and that Jacob would be healthy, but it was not to be. On 7 March 2013 my baby boy was born. Tom and I had three days in intensive care with him. Jacob brought so much love to us in the little time we had. I found myself as a mother, as a woman who cared for someone beyond words. Jacob has, I think, made me a better mother to our twins. I may have two children now, but I truly am the mother of three, something I would not change. I was given a choice and I made the right one for me. People may disagree, but Jacob was my first baby.

When the baby is incompatible with life

A tiny proportion of abortions are carried out in the third trimester (roughly 0.1 per cent in the UK and

1.3 per cent in the US). It's far harder to find reliable statistics for countries where abortion is either severely restricted or banned outright, including the Philippines, Senegal, Egypt and Nicaragua.

Even the most liberal pro-choicers wince at a third-term abortion, but Dr Daniel Grossman, a clinical and public health researcher on abortion and contraception wrote, 'The nerve fibers that connect the pain receptors to the cerebral cortex, where they would be able to perceive the pain, those fibers aren't even present until the third trimester of pregnancy – after twenty-six or twenty-eight weeks.' This isn't 'feeling' or 'I know', it's rigorously researched, evidence-based medicine.

There are three main reasons why a third-term abortion is carried out. Firstly, if the mother did not know that she was pregnant. Secondly, to save the mother's life. And thirdly, because of a catastrophic foetal abnormality. Jacob's mother chose to go through with the pregnancy anyway and to spend three days with him in the ICU.

Another woman might make a different choice. In 2016, the website Jezebel published a deeply moving piece about a woman who discovered early on in her much-wanted pregnancy that there were major problems. They carried on, doing their research and hoping for the best, and then, when she was thirty-one weeks, they found that the baby wouldn't be able to breathe by himself. In the words of the doctor, the baby was 'incompatible with life'. If she went full term, the baby would choke and die. In anguish, she and her husband chose to terminate.

Ayaan

'It has been twenty-five years now, and my
daughter has had her own child, but I am still in
that same bed where I gave birth to her.'

This has been my life since I had my first baby. I married
young and got pregnant right away. My mother had
hoped the blessing of a child would come later, but some
wish for a child for a lifetime and never get the chance,
so I should not complain. The pregnancy was okay. I say
that, as I have nothing to compare it to. I stayed at my
mother's house towards the end. She was scared that
being in the country when the baby came, it might take
the midwife too long to get to me. It was not like
today. There were no phones, let alone mobiles, where
we lived.

I went into labour just after Friday prayer. I remember
like it was yesterday. The house was empty when I began
to feel pain so shocking it took my breath away. I tried
to get off the day bed and saw it was wet, so I knew what
was happening. I waited for someone to come back, and
my little brother was the first. He was nine, and second
was my younger sister, who was eleven. I told him to go
get Mum, our auntie or even our sister. He looked at me,
terrified, like he had seen a ghost, as I was in pain and
my waters were dripping down my legs. He ran and got
my mum from our auntie's house.

My auntie was a birth attendant so, when she hurried

in, I felt some relief, but no break in the pain. Thinking about it, I can still feel the pain, but maybe I really feel the effect it had on my life. I was in labour for almost forty-eight hours. My hips were too small, my auntie said, and her and my mother feared that I would rip and might bleed out. I pushed when she told me and tried not to when she told me to stop. I really did try, but the baby didn't want to come out, and after two days I just wanted it to be over.

I remember pushing so hard I almost passed out and then, finally, hearing Ubah's cry. They took her away and then waited for the afterbirth. There was plastic all over the floor and it was covered in water and blood. I could not smell anything, and I cannot today, but I know there must have been a smell and today I know there is. I stayed at my mum's for forty days, as it's tradition, and being so young I had no idea that it was not normal for my urine to just flow like it did. I seemed to have lost control over my body, as my breasts would leak and as soon as I addressed that I would find I had wet myself. I tried to get up often and pre-empt it, but I just could not.

My mum told me it was normal and it would soon stop. I moved from the bedroom to the back of our small little house to be closer to the toilet.

After forty days the blood stopped, but nothing else did. I had the party to celebrate, but I did not feel like it. I drank nothing for a whole day before and during the party. The idea of sitting down and standing up wet was beyond a nightmare. My husband's family were all coming over and, if they found out what was going on, I was scared they would think I was not worthy of being his wife. I hoped and prayed every day that I would wake up and I would be dry, but it never happened. It has been twenty-five years now and my daughter has had her own child, but I am still in that same bed where I gave birth to her.

When it was time to return to my husband I was more scared than I was as a young bride. I was now a mother, but I was broken, and it would take only moments for him to notice. I begged my mum not to make me go, but she said it would be shameful for me to stay any longer. I remember her looking at me as I leaked on to the hallway tiles.

For the first week it seemed as if maybe things could work, as my husband left me with the baby, and his sister, who was staying with us, did not come into my room. I could clean the floor and bed before anyone noticed, but with Ubah needing to be fed very often I was not able to clean all the mess and in time it began to set in. I had no idea that my condition had a name, or that it was common in the world. I was alone, sixteen years old, with a baby and a house full of people for whom I had no answers. The smell soon took over my room. It was awful when the heat hit, and that is when my mum first said something. She said it was not healthy for Ubah to be in the room, with all the flies and the smell. She would not be able to bring me home, but my younger sister who was not married yet could come and live with me. She would be able to sleep with the baby at night and look after her during the day if I felt I could not leave the room. I really could not say much. I also missed my sister and hoped she would be able to understand, and I could talk to her. We did not talk, but we cried at night and held each other. I think she was also scared and, when someone came for her hand a few weeks later, she refused, and my mother accepted for her, as she saw the fear in her eyes. They also thought I was cursed so, in allowing my sister to get married, people would learn of my illness. I call it 'illness', as that is how I was told to see it until a few weeks ago.

After twenty-five years, while I was visiting my daughter, who was giving birth to her second baby in the capital, I came across the term 'fistula'. This is what I have. I am not ill, it seems, but just have a fixable hole. Don't judge me for crying now, because I know I should be happy, and I am, but I am also so sad. I am so sad that this could have been addressed had I lived in the city or had I visited my daughter when she had her first child three years ago. I could now be a fixed woman. What I am sad about the most, as I await my second grandchild, is that I never had a second child, or even the chance of it. My first pregnancy was my last, the most painful and longest-lasting thing ever in my life. My husband, I am sure you can guess, being a man, went off and had more children of his own. She did not have the issues that I did, and she gave him daughters and sons. I don't hate him for leaving. He married a young woman and expected to be just like his friends, a father to as many kids as God wished for him, a businessman and happy. I am not sure if he is happy, but he is a father to many and did have a business when I last spoke to him.

After the operation I hope you will come back and have tea with me, I will be having a blessing, a celebration, really. I can finally celebrate my pregnancy, my child and being whole again. The forty days of bleeding for me have been years of leaking and now I know why I am thankful to say they are finally over.

Torn apart by childbirth

There are four types of birth tear. The skin around the vagina and the anus – the perineum – is very elastic, but sometimes the baby's head is too large or the skin isn't stretchy enough. Some women have an episiotomy, where the doctor or midwife cuts to prevent a more serious tear. The cut is then sewn back up. Episiotomies used to be quite routine in hospital births, but now it's felt that a natural tear heals better and that episiotomies should only be done if the baby's head is very large or the woman is exhausted from a protracted labour.

First-degree tears are where the skin of the perineum tears. The second degree is when skin *and* muscle tears. Kris, who we heard from earlier, had a third-degree laceration, which is when the skin, muscle and the muscle *up to* the ring of muscle around the anus also tears.

Maureen Treadwell from the Birth Trauma Association

says, 'Women have said it makes them feel dirty, it wrecks their work, their home and their social life. And it's a total taboo.' And these are women in the UK, so the suffering of a young woman like Ayaan in a developing country, without access to medical care, can only be imagined. The hardline natural-childbirth enthusiasts might like to put themselves in Ayaan's position.

Ayaan had the fourth-degree tear, which is where skin, muscle and the ring of muscle around the anus tears. This led to a fistula, or hole, which left her in agony, doubly incontinent and shunned by her family. The Fistula Foundation say that an obstetric fistula is both preventable and treatable, but fewer than six in ten women in developing countries give birth with a trained professional, and they are often very young, their bodies not developed enough for childbirth. Ayaan suffered for twenty-five years, and yet the operation to repair an anal fistula takes about thirty minutes.

Siobhan

'I've never had any issues with my body anyway,
but watching my stomach grow lushly round and
tight and my breasts swell to the size of space
hoppers gave me a profound sense of pleasure.'

My husband and I already had one child and, because I'd had such a terrible time afterwards with severe post-natal depression, we both shut down on the idea of having another. But then suddenly, when I was thirty-eight, my ovaries started smacking me about, so to speak. There's a condition called *Mittelschmerz*, which means 'middle pain' in German. It's a term for ovulation pain, and I had it full on. It would switch from my left side to my right every month and coincided with what I can only describe as a deep, pulling ache to reproduce. Luckily, my husband was equally keen because, at thirty-eight, I really didn't have time to muck about. As the posters in the doctor's office were only too keen to remind me, with a pregnancy arrow plummeting after thirty-five, I would now firmly be defined, in pregnancy terms, as 'geriatric'.

Timing my dates carefully and using my poor husband as a sperm donor ('I'm ovulating. Get your trousers off'), I got pregnant, but I miscarried at twelve weeks. I was told that it could take twelve months for my cycle to return to normal, but I had a strong sense of time running out, so I asked for and was put on a drug called Clomid which pushes your ovaries into pumping out eggs like a mother, and I was pregnant again within three months. I remember taking the test in a stinky pub toilet and crying with joy when a second pale pink line appeared. Now I can't walk by a chemist's and see a First Response pregnancy test without smiling.

I threw up for the first few months, but I didn't mind as my doctor told me that this was a sign the hormones were really whizzing about. And then, in my second trimester, when I felt safe, I began to relax and really enjoy my changing body.

I've never had any issues with my body anyway, but watching my stomach grow lushly round and tight and my breasts swell to the size of space hoppers gave me a profound sense of pleasure. I remember watching the late Robin Williams' *Live at the Met* show, and he had this brilliant section on his wife's pregnancy and how in month five or six 'the titty fairy arrives but the wife turns away, going, "Nope, these are for the baby."' My husband loved my breasts, despite the multitude of blue veins just under the surface. I kept thinking of the London Underground!

After our son was born I struggled with breastfeeding. A baby is born knowing only how to suck, and my God can they suck hard. My poor breasts felt like someone had run a cheese grater over them and, despite everyone telling me how 'natural' it was (that effing word again), I found that one breast only produced a tiny dribble of milk, so I bought an electric breast pump and plugged myself in. It was a revelation, except my nipples tripled in size. I watched, amazed, as the milk squirted into the bottle. It didn't help that my husband stuck his head round the door, making mooing noises.

Breastfeeding

There's a great deal of pressure put on women to breastfeed, often by themselves, but that's not the same as supporting them to do it. The word 'support' is bandied about but, in practical terms, underpaid and overworked hospital midwives are the ones who show exhausted new mothers how to help their baby latch on. Some are brilliant, gently and carefully encouraging and acting as cheerleaders. Others merely jam the nipple against the baby's mouth with all the finesse of getting a household appliance to work.

In the UK currently, only about 30 per cent of babies are still being breastfed after six months, compared to 70 per cent in Norway, with many experts citing an ambivalent attitude to women's bodies being the root cause. They argue that when images of women breastfeeding on social media are routinely taken down because they are deemed 'inappropriate' or even 'taboo' it points towards a misunderstanding of what is 'sexual' and to an ambivalent attitude towards the female body.

From checking round with my friends, a few have openly said that they hated the idea and preferred to bottle feed, but most wanted to breastfeed, but found it more difficult than they had expected. These beatific stock photos of breastfeeding mothers blissfully focused on their babies didn't help. Maybe a few more images of exhausted, wild-eyed mothers and bawling, red-faced infants would help. Siobhan found that once she got past the feeling of being a 'bit like a Jersey cow', as she put it, the electric pump got her milk supply going.

4. The Menopause

'So many women I've talked to see menopause
as an ending. But I've discovered this is your
moment to reinvent yourself after years of
focusing on the needs of everyone else. It's your
opportunity to get clear about what matters to
you and then to pursue that with all of your
energy, time and talent.'
– Oprah Winfrey

'What is the point of being proud of being a
woman if you're going to be desperately
ashamed of this one bit of it – this last third
of your actual life?'
– India Knight, *In Your Prime*

The definition of menopause is 'the period in a woman's
life when menstruation ceases', which, if you grow up
in the West, can be described as the cliff edge of womanhood and, sadly, that's how I've seen it. The final stage
before no-(wo)man's-land, where we are meant to shrivel
up like the Wicked Witch of the West. And what with
the night sweats (probably also with shrieks of 'I'm

melting!'), we watch with a mixture of irritation and sadness as the older man with a young girl is lionized as a 'silver fox', while any woman with a boyfriend younger than her by three months is decreed to have a 'toyboy' or, even worse, be a 'cougar'.

Now, in my thirties, I feel more powerful, confident, sure of myself. I've had enough periods to fill a bath tub and have some idea what is going on down there, I've enjoyed plenty of orgasms, and I look at the way a friend's children play and explore, with that total lack of self-consciousness. I think that *maybe* I might want my own. And my friends who don't want kids, they're clear about it, and unapologetic, as they should be. But overall, I kind of feel like I'm at my peak. Which means there's only one way to go.

We are beginning to talk about it a teeny bit more, but conversation round the menopause is more or less where domestic violence was in the seventies. One or two pockets of bravery (Chiswick Women's Aid, the first ever refuge for battered women, run by Erin Pizzey, since you ask), while the rest of us ignore it or make jokes about the unfeasibly warm weather we're having, while hot-flushing away.

The idea of when middle age begins varies, but many people think of it as a state of mind. 'When you start to discuss your aches and pains and *enjoy it*,' one woman said to me. Another said she realized she was middle-aged when she flicked through a celebrity magazine and couldn't identify a single one. 'I think I managed Katie

Price, but that's it,' she said miserably. But for most women, once the menopause begins, it's a clear sign. You are no longer young.

The menopause doesn't just begin, though. It's preceded by the perimenopause, which can go on for years. Medically, the perimenopause is when the ovaries start to make less oestrogen and your rate of monthly egg drop slows down, but this can begin in your thirties. Suddenly, I don't feel quite so young any more.

Personally, I feel I'll have hit middle age when somebody tells me I look good and I can hear the phrase 'for your age' being bitten back. No wonder it's so difficult for women to feel fanny forward and positive about the menopause – we live in a youth-obsessed culture.

The actor Maggie Gyllenhaal recalled recently being told she was 'too old' at thirty-seven to play the lover of a fifty-five-year-old actor! A perfect example of the gobsmacking sexism that runs through Hollywood, when male actors in their fifties, sixties and beyond are routinely cast opposite female actors in their twenties.

During publicity for the James Bond movie *Spectre*, forty-seven-year-old Daniel Craig was breathlessly questioned about the 'revolutionary addition' of fifty-year-old Monica Bellucci as a Bond girl. 'What's it like succumbing to the charms of an older woman?' asked the interviewer. To his credit, Craig sardonically replied, 'I think you mean the charms of a woman *his own age*.'

If influential women in the film and TV business are furious at being sidelined at the age of forty into a box marked 'old', then what's it like for the rest of us?

When I was thinking about this chapter, I imagined putting out a call:

Perimenopausal and menopausal women, come and talk to me about sex, HRT and being *une femme d'un certain âge.*

I imagined women would come running to tell me their stories, good and bad. When I started the book, I believed that the narrative I'd been sold about the menopause being the end of the world was bullshit. It had to be, with women like the Queen, Hillary Clinton, Angela Merkel, Theresa May, Oprah Winfrey in leading positions in the world. I wanted to show that the menopause wasn't the end – it was the beginning of a new chapter. Sadly, in the Global North, I found this wasn't always the case and, as with much of this book, as soon as I sat down with women and listened, things changed.

I found it hard to talk to women about what it's like when their fertility is gone (sometimes snatched away), or when they feel 'dried up' or invisible, or without the future they envisaged – the wasteland I imagined the menopause to be. I don't want to be the young – well, youngish – fruit looking down on women I respect and love, so, in this chapter more than the others, I've mostly spoken to women I know, women who I can ask the questions I want to and who know I'm not being mean-spirited.

There is still so much shame and fear over women's bodies, and me pointing out that some of the most powerful women in the world are post-menopausal made no difference. If you define yourself, or have been defined by your ability to attract men or be relentlessly fertile, then the menopause really does seem like The End.

My grandmother and many women like her only knew myths and stories, which, to be honest, is the same shit people still write now. That when the menopause 'hits' you are meant to slink off into a corner, not to bother anyone with your hot flushes and insomnia, to dress in loose, baggy clothes because you are No Longer Sexual, and only come out to take care of the grand-children.

But as journalist and writer India Knight writes in *In Your Prime*, 'What is the point of being proud of being a woman if you're going to be desperately ashamed of this one bit of it – this last third of your actual life?'

Kara

'In one fell swoop I went from (what I thought I
was) fecund and youthful to a post-menopausal
old lady.'

When I was twenty-nine I had what seemed to be the longest period of my life. Although there was no pain, it just went on and on, a first day of period Groundhog Day. I'd just moved to New York for work, though, so I put it down to stress and a new job. After eleven days, it was still like day one, so, worried, I went to a walk-in clinic a few blocks down. I still remember the wide-eyed shock on the doctor's face as I lay with my legs hoisted.

This doctor literally ran out, returning a minute later with two other doctors. They all gathered round the non-speaking end and gazed in silence. I don't know why I felt embarrassed, but it was the most awkward moment of my life – in a cold room, flat on my back, legs in stirrups and three doctors all staring at my fanny with expressions as though they'd found a giant squid up there. I did consider making a joke, just to break the silence, but I was too busy working out if I should close my legs or not. Sadly, what they found wasn't the alien squid from *Men in Black* (which I could have coped with) but something much nastier – cancer. It seemed that, since my last smear, a few months before I left for NYC, a growth had appeared. I was religious about getting smears, so it seemed insanely unfair. The bleeding, which I thought was just my period, was the early sign of ovarian cancer.

When the doctor told me, I was still lying on my back in this bright, cold doctor's room. Would it have made any difference if I were sitting up? No better, perhaps, but there's something uniquely passive and submissive about lying there, afraid and vulnerable, while the medical profession towers over you like God. There is something about lying on your back while hearing devastating news that puts you at a disadvantage – the passive patient. Maybe I was in shock, but I couldn't believe what I was hearing or how far I was from everyone I knew.

I was told I needed surgery right away, as in, immediately. I could have the operation there and then, which would mean that the bleeding would stop or, if I could get a flight back to the UK, it would need to be done within the week. I chose to have surgery there, honestly thinking it would be a matter of removing the growth and that would be it. Once the surgeons went in, though, it was worse than they expected; the cancer had spread and I would need a hysterectomy. I was not even thirty and I was facing losing my womb, losing the chance to have children and hitting menopause. Well, I would just be post-menopausal; it wouldn't be a gradual process with time to adjust, there would be no stages and no conversation. I had to have the hysterectomy and, overnight, any cosy imaginings of babies at some time vanished. Gone. In one fell swoop I went from (what I thought I was) fecund and youthful to a post-menopausal old lady. I don't look it and, even if people know, they seem to think it is not the same. I zoomed past my mother, who was in her sixties and had been 'going through the change for ten years'. In less than ten hours I was right at the end, just like my grandmother, who had passed away a few years before. I wasn't just dried up, I was completely empty – devoid of eggs. I know that, without the hysterectomy, the cancer may well have killed me, but I didn't even have time to freeze some of my eggs. Choosing not to have a child is one thing, and up to that point I wasn't sure, but to know there is absolutely no possibility was so painful. I desperately needed support.

When I woke up, my head thick from the anaesthetic, my mother was sitting by my bed. She looked at me and said, 'Well, I guess the idea of me having grandchildren is gone.' I closed my eyes and felt tears trickling down my face. My youth was gone, I would have no children – ever. Instead I'd have hot flushes, mood swings and a useless, selfish mother.

Sudden menopause

If you're a man reading this, firstly, kudos; secondly, well done for making it to the menopause section; and thirdly, well . . . imagine being told that you have a choice. You can either die or have a chemical castration, and you have only a few hours to make up your mind. Because, quite reasonably, you want to live, you decide on the latter. Next day, you wake up and the full realization of what's happened washes over you. It might still be possible to get an erection, says the doctor, but you probably won't care if you do because there's not a lot of testosterone left. Oh, and you might also get hot flushes. But hey – you're alive.

As well as waking up to this, Kara also had to deal with a selfish, possibly narcissistic mother who thought only of her lack of grandchildren.

Diane Danzebrink, writing in the *Telegraph*, had a similar experience to Kara. Even though she was a psychotherapist with medical menopause training, she underwent a hysterectomy, which is the surgical removal of the uterus, plus removal of her ovaries. While in hospital she was given no information about the effects of her surgery, even though her body was punched into immediate menopause. She went to her GP and turned down HRT. Her GP didn't ask her why or explain that there are different types, or that the sudden dramatic loss of oestrogen might cause symptoms such as depression, insomnia and anxiety. Months later, after struggling with all three, her husband took her back to the GP after she admitted thinking seriously about suicide. This time, they had a productive conversation and she accepted HRT, which eased her symptoms.

The National Institute for Health and Care Excellence (NICE) produced guidelines for health professionals on the menopause in 2015, but many GPs admit to never having read them. The menopause can be difficult enough, but when it happens suddenly, the shock compounds the lack of care or even interest. Diane went on to campaign for better advice and care for menopausal women. 'It's no joking matter,' she writes. Figures produced by the Samaritans say women between the ages of fifty and fifty-four have the highest suicide rate per 100,000 in the UK.

The average age of menopause is fifty-one.

Maria

'I wanted freedom and that is what
I have now, at last.'

I am sixty-six years old and the menopause has freed me. Many see it as taking away all that is female, which it has, but being female is what has held me hostage all my life.

I was circumcised at fourteen and then, days later, I was married off to a man who was not much younger than I am today. I was his fifth wife and he paid my father in forty cows and home-made beer, a handsome price. Before I became his wife, I hadn't set eyes on him. I married a stranger. It was bad at the beginning, but every girl goes through this, so I had to find a way to get used to it. I was the gift of youth that neither he nor his other wives had. I remember looking at the children running around and the old women in the corner who were older than my mother now, who were to be my sister wives. I had no idea about what being married or being a mother would mean. Now, looking back, I'm glad nobody told me.

I knew he had a lot of money and he wanted more children, and I was his ticket. He paid for me with cows and beer and now I had to produce babies for this old man. But the older I became and the more I saw, the more I hated my youth, my periods and my body. I wished so much to be like my brothers, to be a person. Instead, I was a useful thing, a shell containing what men wanted. I wanted freedom and that is what I have now, at last.

I became pregnant very quickly and, every year for the next ten years, I would be pregnant again and again. Of course, this filled my husband and his family with joy. But I was filled with horror every single time. I knew what was coming. I would look at his first and second wife and wish desperately to be like them. I prayed for the burden of womanhood to be taken away from me, that I would not be hands deep in the blood and pain of my youth. And when I was not pregnant I would bleed for days at a time. As I was the youngest wife and my children were only babies, it was me that had to wash the bloody clothes and the babies' nappies. I paid over and over for those forty cows and home-made beer, for sure, and my reward is only now being cashed in.

Giving birth when you have had FGM is so painful. Maybe it's not so bad if you have a doctor, but I didn't have one, or any pain relief. I had a midwife with a knife. The passage where the baby is meant to pass was too small for every one of my ten babies, and the midwife would cut me as much as she had to, like a can opener. We get tinned food occasionally and we open it with a knife. I used to see my mother struggling to open the can, and that is what crossed my mind as they were opening me to deliver my first baby. Hearing my baby cry as I lay in agony, fighting for my life, was the only thing that brought me back. I think that is why I did not die. I knew that I could not leave my children.

But I survived and now, at sixty-six, I eat well and am at peace. I am blessed I have not developed fistula, so my bladder keeps its urine. When I was forty-five I started to have my period once every few months. I had three in the year I turned fifty, but about ten years ago my periods stopped completely. My daughters are old enough to wash my rags, but there is no need for it. I am meant to cry and long for the blood, the youth and being wanted. But I don't. My husband passed away a long time ago and, in my culture, as his family's property, his younger brother inherited me and my children. He had a younger wife, so when I joined his family I was left alone for a while. But back then my period was still a calling card. My fertility drove male desire and it was what I hated the most.

In this stage of my life I should be begging the gods to be wanted and not to be left out for the dogs. That is what is meant to happen. If I am not worth any cows or home-made beer, not wanted by a man or cannot have kids, I should be left out for the dogs like a dying cow. We did that when I was growing up. If a cow became ill or had a sick calf, if the boys could not carry it back they would leave it for the dogs to eat. I have been left for the dogs, but the dogs have not come for me. Instead, I have found peace. I have found the end of abuse. I sit here today, surrounded by many who feel sorry for me but have no idea how happy I am.

There is no pain or fear in this stage of my life, just milk, butter and peace. I will tell my daughters not to fear this stage but to look forward to it. Of course, they fear it now, they fear not being wanted and being replaced by someone younger. Men will always seek fresher fruit, but this is their own burden and they should be pitied for it. The menopause frees us from the rubbish of the world, but nothing frees men but death.

Amina

'I had no idea that being menopausal would hit
me so hard. Even saying the word chokes me
with grief.'

I am hopeless, miserable and I am taking every day as it comes. I know things are different and I should accept it. But I just can't. I don't want to fall off the edge and become invisible. I don't want to lose what little it seems I have. I have always been visible. I'm an only child, I'm tall and I was always what men wanted. When I started to miss periods I was in my late thirties and working on a big deal, so I blamed it on the stress, but at the back of my mind I knew what it really was. My family has a history of early-onset menopause and my mother was only in her forties when she went through 'the change', as she and millions still call it. I was dating a man I kind of liked, but he was an artist and I wasn't willing to settle. Perhaps I should have, as 'not settling' has got me where I am today, alone and scared. When I realized, I called my best friend, but decided to go to the clinic alone. Although I'm very close to my mum, I couldn't bear to ask her to come with me to a doctor for the hormone test that would confirm what I knew was happening. The fear I felt going in, the knowledge that the life I thought I had, my plans for children – knowing that all that would be at risk, so much rested on that test. I was three weeks shy of my fortieth, I had an amazing job, a flat in Manhattan and the world still ahead of me, or so I thought, but I came out of that doctor's appointment knowing that I might never have kids, I was never going to be the woman I wanted to be, and it hurt so bad. I stood outside the clinic and just broke down. My vision of the future was lost.

I'm not saying that the menopause is like cancer, but

I've seen friends crumple at a cancer diagnosis, not just because they had a serious illness, it's more seeing their health and life just disappear in front of them. That's what I felt. My future was gone in a puff of hormones. I didn't tell anyone and, as soon as I got home that night, I drank a bottle of vodka and hit the town with my friend. She thought I just needed to party it off, but I wanted to prove the doctor wrong and get pregnant. I fucked everyone I knew in my phonebook and anyone I could pick up. I went from being picky to being needy. This soon made the men run a mile. They could smell the fear and desperation. And despite all the sex, I felt more and more empty, my heart was broken and my soul was screaming but no one could hear. I had no idea that being menopausal would hit me so hard. Even saying the word chokes me with grief. My periods stopped a full three years ago. I haven't been taking any medication, as I don't trust any of this shit they have. I don't care that my vagina is dry, as I don't have a sex drive anyway. I can't bear to look at myself, let alone think a man would look at me.

I used to complain about not being able to walk down the street without men catcalling me, but now the silence is deafening. At parties I can stand at the bar waiting for a drink where, before, my cup was never empty, literally or metaphorically.

My cup will be empty from now on, and I know I need to accept this, so I'm getting help. I hope I can feel some acceptance and peace soon. If you look around the city I live in, many women my age will be projecting a happy and full life. They're either my age or older. They don't have kids or someone in their beds, but they seem happy. Or maybe they're just busy. But it's all bullshit anyway. We live in a youth-obsessed world so the women drying up are not the river anyone wants to drink from. I don't know what my role in life is now. It's not as if my job is about saving the world. I haven't given much to the community or to people around me. I love my mum and dad, but they are getting old, and I don't have any siblings. I am alone, and that is scary. I feel myself ageing, and I hate it. I don't want to die in a room all alone. I hope that I find some purpose soon and die doing something exciting, or be really New York and get hit by a bus while crossing the road. But there is so much traffic I'll probably just get yelled at, and a couple of broken bones. I might not even mind being shouted at, as at least someone will be seeing me.

I'm sorry to be so dark, but I'm in a dark place and this is my experience. I hope you either enjoy your life now or that, when you are hit with the change, the world is a better place for women.

When it's too late to have children

Singer Janet Jackson gave birth a few weeks short of her fiftieth birthday. Geena Davis had her first baby at forty-six and her twins at forty-eight. What do these women have in common? Shedloads of cash and access to the best obstetricians money can buy. Sorry to be crude, but it's the truth. It costs between $10,000 and $30,000 to have an uncomplicated delivery in the US, so fertility treatments can be eye-wateringly expensive. Of course, we don't see that – just a gorgeous woman with her babies. So, it's not surprising that we're sometimes a bit hazy about when time is really running out.

A stark reminder is when you look at a fertility chart and realize that, for most women, it drops like a stone after the age of thirty-five. You can, however, have a fertility MOT, which isn't as hideous as it sounds. (I have this terrible vision of a mechanic looking at my undercarriage and going, 'Nah, this is a clapped-out old banger.') It's a blood test which determines how many eggs you have left. But doctors have pointed out that what this test *doesn't* determine is the *quality* of your eggs. It's so bloody unfair. Men can carry on shagging and producing well into their eighties. Only the other day I read of seventy-year-old Ronnie Wood (cue the Paul Merton gag – 'His hairstyle is older than his girlfriend') and his cute twin girls. And yet when Dr Patricia Rashbrook, a child psychologist, had an IVF baby at sixty-two, she was 'selfish' and it was 'absurd'.

Sinead

'With the menopause, it was different – more like a flat, colourless landscape.'

My mother's generation had a different attitude to the menopause. She had a different attitude, full stop. My boyfriend was hoovering once, and she followed him round her house, her face shining with wonder, as though he'd just split the atom.

Mum was Catholic and had a habit of offering up pain for 'her sins' instead of going to a doctor, unfortunately. She truly believed that her easy menopause was because God took pity on her after giving her wretchedly painful periods. 'Didn't feel a thing,' she'd say, while glaring purse-lipped at my dusty shelves. (I've always been a working mother.)

My mother died very suddenly, just as my own menopause was kicking in. And kick it did, probably because not only had I never made any deals with God, I'd also renounced Catholicism and gone on numerous pro-choice marches. I could cope with the hot flushes and bouts of insomnia, but there was one day when I was sitting and the sunlight from my garden was pouring in, and I just felt . . . flat. As though all the joy in my life had just oozed out. And no matter how sternly I reminded myself that my life was great, in that I had enjoyable work and great friends, and healthy children and blah blah blah . . . I still felt grey.

The Australian psychologist Dorothy Rowe has written several wonderful books on depression, and one of the most helpful sections is when she suggests you describe your depression as a physical thing. When I had post-natal depression, it was a sense of being frozen and immobile. With the menopause, it was different – more like a flat, colourless landscape. I took this landscape to my doctor, who explained about the fluctuating levels of oestrogen and progesterone. It's no one-size-fits-all, so some women need to have their treatment adjusted, but I was given an HRT patch, which worked very quickly. I couldn't believe how much better I felt – it was like the sun coming out.

The 'M' word

In 2018, Leicester University introduced a menopause policy. It suggested that women might need a fan to cool down when having hot flushes or have flexible working hours to cope with insomnia. Of course, the media hit on Dr Andrea Davies's semi-jokey suggestion for male colleagues to say 'menopause' three times a day to normalize the word. The *Daily Mail* covered the story, complete with a helpful stock photo of a woman wearing a pained expression and holding one hand to her head while another grasped a mini-fan. Meanwhile, the comments ranged from 'I thought we employed intelligent people at universities!' to one annoyed man suggesting, 'Well, women should shout "Impotence" three times a day' in solidarity with men.

Magda

'It takes years of living to really accept yourself,
lines and bags and all.'

I don't see why women are so afraid of the menopause. Of course, if you're feeling seriously depressed, anxious or sweating buckets, then I have every sympathy and these symptoms need to be taken seriously but, my goodness, look at the upside. A hundred years ago, you'd be some old crone, if you were still alive. Now, your kids are (hopefully, dear God) independent, and you no longer have to worry about getting pregnant. You have years ahead of you, in which to learn new things, have sex, travel. And now you'll enjoy them even more because you have life experience.

My children are grown up and, while I love to see them, they have their own lives. My son got a bit cross with me the other day because he wanted to have coffee and I've got so much on I couldn't see him for a few weeks!

I'm divorced and live on my own – very happily, thank you. I've got a boyfriend, but we don't live together. It started out that way because he has a house about fifty miles from me, but I needed to stay where I was to keep close to my children's father. Now the children have grown up, I've discovered I like solitude. It also means that when my boyfriend and I meet up we make more of an effort.

You want to know about the sex, don't you? Well, I've stayed fit but still put on weight, alas. But my boyfriend adores my body. I went through a period of vaginal dryness but there are loads of lubes out there. Although I did accidentally once overuse a small pot of tiger balm after some fool who shall remain nameless (my boyfriend) said he'd read somewhere that it intensified orgasm if you put a little on to the clitoris. I used too much and it was like a chili explosion in my pants.

When I was younger and more beautiful, I didn't realize it. I truly believe young women are sold a crock by the beauty industry and the diet industry. They wouldn't make any money if they really meant you should accept yourself or be comfortable in your own skin. It takes years of living to really accept yourself, lines and bags and all. Of course, I sometimes glance at my face in a harsh light and realize that, although I may feel twenty-one inside, I'm not. I'm a woman in my fifties. I have lines. I get hot flushes. I will never be able to idly trace my fingers over my jutting hipbones again.

And yet . . .

I wouldn't want to be back in my teens or twenties if you paid me a million quid, really. Yes, I'd have firm flesh and a line-free face, but I'd also be skittering about not knowing who I was, wishing I looked like anybody other than me, oh so anxious about connecting with the world and my place in it. I put up with so much bloody nonsense from men, too. As Helen Mirren said, 'If I could give my younger self one piece of advice it would be to use the words "fuck off" much more frequently.'

Middle-aged women – we need you!

This is not a joke. Really. Younger women need not apply. After a three-year investigation into the intelligence services, a government report recommended they recruit more middle-aged women, because they are more 'emotionally intelligent and intuitive'. 'Try Mumsnet', added the report, *taps side of nose*. Mumsnet users immediately rose to the challenge, pointing out that 'parents have eyes in the back of their head anyway'. Charlotte33 was convinced of her suitability as she had 'an amazing gut instinct for tosspots'. What this government report left out, however, was a middle-aged woman's greatest asset, her self-proclaimed invisibility. As one Mumsnetter snarked, 'I'd make a great spy. I go totally unnoticed everywhere I go, but I have a keen eye for detail. Nobody suspects a woman in Mum boots of *anything* underhand.'

Conclusion

'Sigmund Freud once asked, "What do women
want?" before proceeding to tell them. He was
the founder of both psychoanalysis
and mansplaining.'

         – Anonymous

We want pretty much the same as men. Once we get past Maslow's basic needs of food, water, shelter and half-decent broadband, we all want to feel safe and loved. We also want to do something with our lives, whether it's to be an astronaut, or raise a family, or write a book, or live solo. But to achieve any kind of potential we need to be in charge of our own bodies and at peace within them. We might be a Somali or Egyptian girl at risk from FGM, or a young woman in El Salvador afraid to report a miscarriage for fear of being jailed for the 'crime' of abortion. Or the outwardly privileged woman with her longed-for baby who guiltily remembers her life before twenty-four-hour milking duty, or the forty-five-year-old woman who feels as though all colour has been leached from her life, as well as her hair.

We're not all prisoners of our femaleness, but we all share the rites of passage that make us female. Some, we can choose to circumvent, depending where we live. And there's no doubt that the life of a well-educated, moneyed woman in the West is going to be light years removed from that of a woman in a refugee camp or a girl who is bought for marriage. This is a book about the fanny, however, and not poverty, although the two, sadly, often go together.

But there is validation in shared experience. And sheer bloody relief. Women have always shared intimate details. A man glancing at a group of women howling with laughter over a bottle of wine might well shiver because, yes, they probably *are* discussing how crap their exes were in bed. And later, after another bottle, they'll share puking and pooing birth stories. A man, on the other hand, can work with another man for forty years and not know if he even has kids.

Changes happen incrementally, both good and bad. The year 2017 saw the first Bodyform campaign using red liquid. The following year saw the first attempt, in Somalia, of an FGM prosecution, and Ireland repealing the Eighth Amendment, which now means Irish women can get an abortion up to twelve weeks. But at the same time, in the US reproductive rights are being chipped away. Globally, what the changes and setbacks have in common is the theme of women's bodies plus secrecy and shame. The more women discuss our commonality, the less of a hold those twin monsters, secrecy and shame, have on us.

Acknowledgements

This book would not have been possible without the incredible women who were brave enough to talk openly with me. Some of you are dear friends I have known for years and others are women I only met once but who will for ever be my heroes. I love and respect each and every one of you, the world seeks to divide but we are united in our commitment to keep speaking up and out.

I would also like to thank editors Emily Robertson and Jane Purcell. Emily, thank you for being so patient as I found the strength to write this book. We have both grown since we met and I am so thankful for you and all your support, and Jane, thank you for giving me the confidence to trust my words and supporting me to see that my words had value. I am fanny grateful for you both.